DRUGS AND THE KIDNEY

Other titles in the *New Clinical Applications* Series:

Dermatology (Series Editor Dr J.L. Verbov)
Dermatological Surgery
Superficial Fungal Infections
Talking Points in Dermatology – I
Treatment in Dermatology
Current Concepts in Contact Dermatitis
Talking Points in Dermatology – II
Tumours, Lymphomas and Selected Paraproteinaemias
Relationships in Dermatology
Talking Points in Dermatology – III
Mycobacterial Skin Diseases

Rheumatology (Series Editors Dr J.J. Calabro† and Dr W. Carson Dick)
Ankylosing Spondylitis
Infections and Arthritis

Nephrology (Series Editor Professor G.R.D. Catto)
Continuous Ambulatory Peritoneal Dialysis
Management of Renal Hypertension
Chronic Renal Failure
Calculus Disease
Pregnancy and Renal Disorders
Haemodialysis
Multisystem Diseases
Urinary Tract Infection
Transplantation
Glomerulonephritis
Drugs and the Kidney

NEW
CLINICAL
APPLICATIONS
NEPHROLOGY

DRUGS AND THE KIDNEY

Editor
G.R.D. CATTO
MD, DSc, FRCP, FRCP (Lond., Edin. and Glasg.)
Professor of Medicine
University of Aberdeen
UK

KLUWER ACADEMIC PUBLISHERS
DORDRECHT / BOSTON / LONDON

Distributors

for the United States and Canada: Kluwer Academic Publishers, PO Box 358, Accord Station, Hingham, MA 02018–0358, USA
for all other countries: Kluwer Academic Publishers Group, Distribution Center, PO Box 322, 3300 AH Dordrecht, The Netherlands

British Library Cataloguing in Publication Data

Drugs and the kidney.
1. Man. Kidneys. Diseases caused by drugs
I. Catto, Graeme R.D. (Graeme Robertson Dawson), *1945–*
II. Series
616′.6′1071

Library of Congress Cataloging-in-Publication Data

Drugs and the kidney/editor, G.R.D. Catto.
p. cm.–(New clinical applications. Nephrology)
Includes bibliographical references.

ISBN-13: 978-94-010-7624-1 e-ISBN-13: 978-94-009-2492-5

DOI: 10.1007/978-94-009-2492-5

1. Kidneys–Effect of drugs on. 2. Drugs–Side effects.
I. Catto, Graeme R.D. II. Series.
[DNLM: 1. Analgesics–adverse effects. 2. Anti-Inflammatory Agents, Non-Steroidal–pharmacology. 3. Kidney–drug effects. 4. Kidney–physiology. 5. Monitoring Physiologic. 6. Nephritis, Interstitial–chemically induces. WJ 300 D7941]
RC903.9.D78 1989
616.6′1–dc20
DNLM/DLC
for Library of Congress 89–24593
CIP

Published in the United Kingdom by Kluwer Academic Publishers, PO Box 55, Lancaster, UK.

Kluwer Academic Publishers BV incorporates the publishing programmes of D. Reidel, Martinus Nijhoff, Dr W. Junk and MTP Press.

CONTENTS

LIST OF AUTHORS

P. Kincaid-Smith
Department of Nephrology
Royal Melbourne Hospital
Parkville
Victoria 3050
Australia

F.P. Marsh
Renal Unit
The London Hospital
Whitechapel
London E1 1BB
UK

C.G. Newstead
Renal Unit
The London Hospital
Whitechapel
London E1 1BB
UK

A.K. Scott
Department of Pharmacology
and Therapeutics
University of Liverpool
Ashton Street, PO Box 147
Liverpool L69 3BX
UK

J.A. Vale
West Midlands Poisons Unit
Dudley Road Hospital
Birmingham B18 7QH
UK

SERIES EDITOR'S FOREWORD

In recent years both doctors and patients have become increasingly aware that many essential drugs may induce unfortunate side-effects in susceptible individuals. The kidney is the principal route of excretion for many of these substances and may as a result become involved in pathological processes. Developments in haemodialysis and haemoperfusion may be of value in increasing the rate of excretion of potentially toxic substances but it is essential that the advantages and disadvantages of these techniques are fully appreciated by all with an interest in clinical practice.

This book details the recent advances in understanding of analgesic nephropathy, interstitial nephritis, elimination of poisons and drug monitoring. Each chapter has been written by a recognized expert in the field and provides information of relevance and practical importance to the average clinician. The developments of the last decade have emphasized that drug toxicity is a subject on which all clinicians, but perhaps especially nephrologists, should be fully informed.

ABOUT THE EDITOR

Professor Graeme R.D. Catto is Professor in Medicine and Therapeutics at the University of Aberdeen and Honorary Consultant Physician/Nephrologist to the Grampian Health Board. His current interest in transplant immunology was stimulated as a Harkness Fellow at Harvard Medical School and the Peter Bent Brighton Hospital, Boston, USA. He is a member of many medical societies including the Association of Physicians of Great Britain and Ireland, the Renal Association and the Transplantation Society. He has published widely on transplant and reproductive immunology, calcium metabolism and general nephrology.

1

ANALGESIC NEPHROPATHY AND THE EFFECT OF NON-STEROIDAL ANTI-INFLAMMATORY DRUGS ON THE KIDNEY

P. KINCAID-SMITH

INTRODUCTION

The chronic nephrotoxicity associated with excessive use of over-the-counter analgesic mixtures and compounds was recognized some 25 years before the documentation of the acute syndromes of renal failure and the nephrotic syndrome attributed to pharmacological doses of non-steroidal anti-inflammatory drugs (NSAIDs). Spuhler and Zollingers' description[1] in 1953 of chronic interstitial nephritis in patients taking excessive amounts of phenacetin-containing mixtures was the first documentation of what has become known as analgesic nephropathy. Papers describing the acute nephrotoxicity of NSAIDs first appeared in the late 1970s although they have increased considerably in number over the past 10 years.

Controversy originally surrounded the question as to whether pharmacological doses of NSAIDs taken over a period of years can also cause the chronic lesions of papillary necrosis[2] and irreversible chronic renal failure[3]. This observation provides a link between the nephrotoxicity of NSAIDs and analgesic nephropathy – especially since aspirin, itself an NSAID, is an important ingredient of compound analgesic preparations in many countries and has sometimes been the only drug implicated as a cause of renal papillary necrosis[4].

Because the mechanisms involved in nephrotoxicity are probably quite separate in the acute syndrome and in the chronic lesions of renal papillary necrosis, these two conditions will be discussed separately.

ANALGESIC NEPHROPATHY AND CHRONIC RENAL PAPILLARY NECROSIS ASSOCIATED WITH NSAIDs

Historical

Spuhler and Zollinger[1] first described chronic interstitial nephritis in a group of patients who had taken excessive quantities of phenacetin-containing analgesic mixtures. They noted a yellowish, flaky appearance of the papilla in 16 of 29 cases and suggested that these papillary lesions were secondary to the cortical lesion of chronic interstitial nephritis which they considered to be both the major and the primary lesion.

Over the next decade reports of renal papillary necrosis associated with excessive use of a variety of over-the-counter analgesic compounds and mixtures appeared from Scandinavia, Canada and Australia. It is of interest, in view of recent experimental findings with caffeine, that, wherever analgesic nephropathy has posed a problem in the community, caffeine-containing analgesic powders have been implicated as the major cause of the renal damage.

The clinical syndrome associated with analgesic nephropathy emerged in many countries around the middle of this century and is now rapidly declining following the introduction of measures to restrict availability of the relevant over-the-counter medications.

Studies of the autopsy prevalence of renal papillary necrosis from several European countries and from Australia showed an increasing prevalence (Table 1.1). The alarming prevalence in Australia revealed in studies in New South Wales, which documented renal papillary necrosis in as many as 20% of all autopsies only a decade ago, was ten times as high as that recorded in Denmark, 20 times as high as Switzerland and almost 100 times that recorded at autopsy in the United Kingdom at about the same time.

No recent study of autopsy prevalence has been carried out in Australia but the clinical syndrome has become rare and there is a steady decline in the number of patients presenting with end-stage

TABLE 1.1 Incidence (%) of analgesic nephropathy in different countries

Australia		
Jacobs and Morris (1962)	Sydney	3.7
Burry (1966)	Brisbane	7.0
Nanra (1968)	Melbourne	8.7
Arnold (1973)	Sydney	21.4
Burry (1977)	Brisbane	8.6
Denmark		
Schourop (1951)		0.2
Schourup (1955)		2.5
Kjaerulff and Harvald (1968)		2.8
Switzerland		
Gloor (1938–1947)		0.76
Gloor (1948–1955)		1.32
Gsell		1.75
New Zealand		
Burry (1974)		1.6
England		
Davies (1961)		0.07
Davies (1967)		0.38
Cove-Smith and Knapp (1978)		0.41
Scotland		
Boyd (1964)		0.60
USA		
Heptinstall (1947–1961)		0.23

(Reproduced from Ref. 139)

renal failure due to analgesic nephropathy (Figure 1.1). This decline is attributed to restriction of sales of over-the-counter analgesics mixtures between 1979 and 1980.

Pathology

In discussing the pathology of analgesic nephropathy it is important to consider the relationship between the lesion of chronic interstitial nephritis and that of renal papillary necrosis.

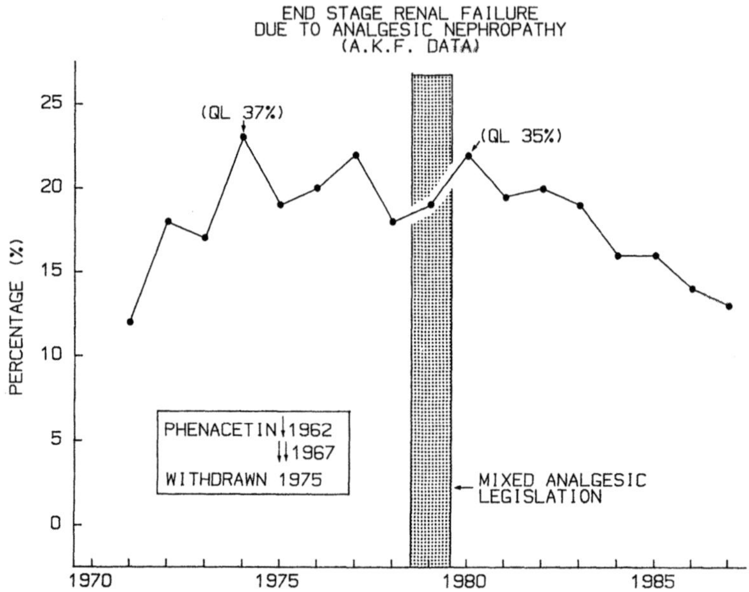

FIGURE 1.1 Patients presenting for treatment of end-stage renal failure in Australia, 1970–1987.

The shaded area indicates time during which legislation limiting over-the-counter sales was introduced. The prevalence of cases with analgesic nephropathy appears to be falling steadily in spite of a progressive increase in mean age of patients accepted for treatment.

Availability of phenacetin decreased considerably in 1962 and it was removed from one of two remaining over-the-counter drugs in 1969 and from the last one in 1975

Spuhler and Zollinger[1] made little of the papillary lesion and their view that it was secondary to chronic interstitial nephritis was readily accepted by Scandinavian workers at that time[5,6]. Previous authors describing other types of papillary necrosis had also concluded that the papillary lesions were secondary to the cortical lesions[7,8].

The clinical observations that patients first presenting with analgesic nephropathy may have normal-sized kidneys with histologically normal renal cortex and that the shrinkage of the kidney which follows separation of papillae is associated with the development of the atrophic cortical lesions of so-called chronic interstitial nephritis support the view that the lesion of renal papillary necrosis is the primary one[9]. While there was some resistance to acceptance of this view when it was first put forward[10,11], it is now generally accepted that renal papillary necrosis precedes so-called chronic interstitial nephritis. Support for this view comes from experimental renal papillary necrosis[12]. In kidneys, from animals receiving various analgesic mixtures, papillary necrosis appears while the overlying cortex is normal. Subsequently, features of cortical atrophy appear in areas drained by tubules obstructed in the necrotic process in the papilla. This sequence of events establishes beyond doubt that cortical changes in this form of experimental papillary necrosis are the consequence of the papillary lesion. Davies[13] had documented a similar sequence of events in experimental papillary necrosis produced in rabbits by ethylenimine and Lucke *et al.*[14] have described similar cortical changes following removal of the renal papilla. These experimental investigations and two independent Australian studies in human kidneys led to acceptance of the view that the papillary lesion is the primary event which results in the secondary cortical changes of so-called chronic interstitial nephritis[9,15].

Analgesic nephropathy is a chronic form of renal papillary necrosis contrasting with the more acute lesions, which are often a preterminal event in diabetes and other forms of renal papillary necrosis. Characteristically there are episodes in which separation of papillae occurs and patients may continue to pass papillary tissue in the urine over many years.

The renal lesions seen in Australia probably differ to some extent from those seen in Europe; Figure 1.2 shows a typical example of the lesion seen in Australia. Characteristic atrophic cortex is seen over necrotic papillae. The cortex in the so-called columns of Bertin is hypertrophied. These lesions produce horizontal bars of hypertrophy on the outer surface of the kidney. The papillae are deeply pigmented and the whole papilla tends to separate and leave a large papillary cavity. In European cases the papilla is more likely to remain attached and to show multiple small areas of necrosis or so-called medullary cavities (Figure 1.3). While separation is the usual feature seen in Australian cases of renal papillary necrosis, the papilla may remain attached and cause some difficulty in the radiological diagnosis[16].

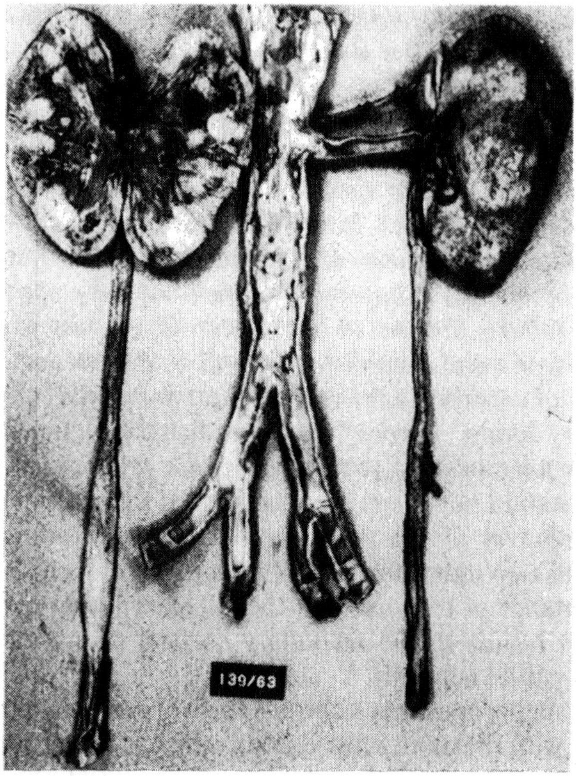

FIGURE 1.2 Cut surface of the right kidney and outer surface of the left kidney in a case of analgesic nephropathy.

The cut surface shows pale areas of hypertrophy in Bertin's columns which are represented by horizontal bars of hypertrophy on the outer surface. Black pigmented papillae are seen in two upper calyces. There is extensive atheroma in this 44-year-old man, another feature associated with analgesic nephropathy

In renal papillary necrosis occurring as a chronic lesion in association with pharmacological doses of NSAIDs, pigmentation is absent and the so-called *in situ* necrosis occurs without separation of the papilla. The same features are seen in analgesic nephropathy occurring in Australia following the withdrawal of phenacetin. In such cases, patients taking aspirin or aspirin combined with one or more of paracetamol, salicylamide or caffeine develop papillary necrosis in

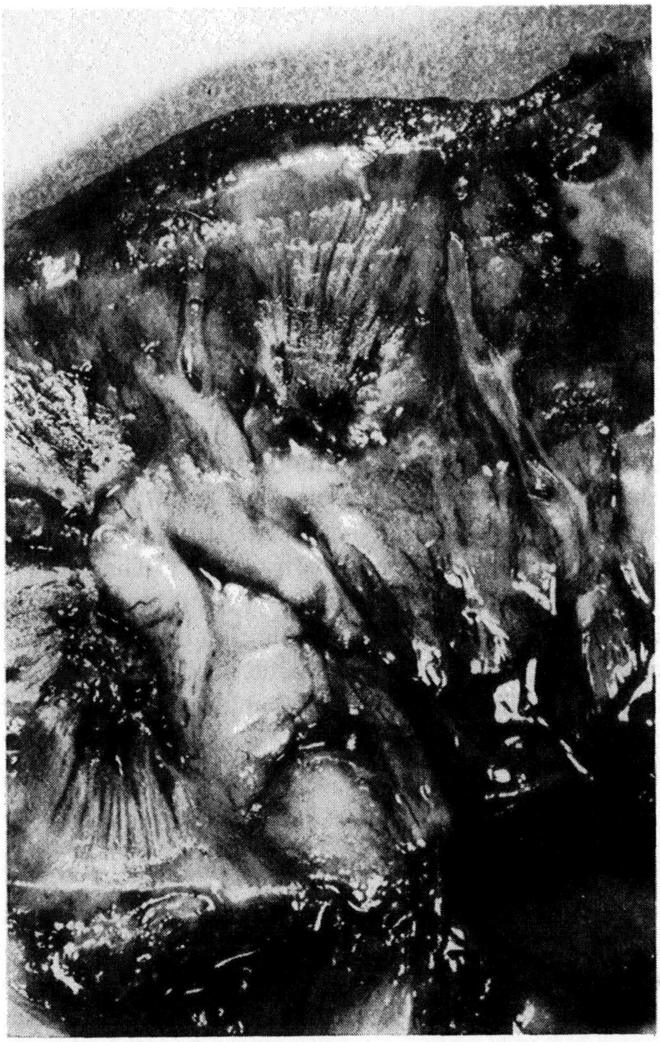

FIGURE 1.3 Cut surface of kidney showing multiple small cavities within the papilla in a case of analgesic nephropathy from Switzerland. These cavities occur where necrotic papillary tissue has separated

not pigmented and is more likely to remain attached than to separate. Calcification commonly occurs within the necrotic papilla and metaplastic bone formation may occur.

Microscopic features

Microscopic examination of the cortex shows only oedema and streaky inflammatory cell infiltration in the acute stages, when recent necrosis of the related papilla has occurred.

In chronic cases, the major features are tubular atrophy and interstitial fibrosis with some interstitial cellular infiltration but a relatively non-specific appearance may be observed in atrophic areas. In Bertin's columns, marked hypertrophy of glomeruli and tubules is present with little or no cellular infiltration or interstitial fibrosis. Within the papilla itself, Burry[15,17] has described a number of early and intermediate changes which precede frank necrosis.

Thickening of the wall and of the interstitial tissue around vasa recta has been noted microscopically by Gloor[18]. This lesion is similar to that described in experimental analgesic nephropathy[19]. Concentric thickening of the wall of small vessels in the urothelium has recently been described in patients with analgesic nephropathy. This may be valuable in providing a diagnosis of analgesic nephropathy from bladder biopsies[20].

Epidemiology and prevalence

The very variable prevalence of analgesic nephropathy in different countries (Table 1.1) and even within countries seems to depend upon the type of over-the-counter analgesic available and the amounts consumed by the population in different areas. Murray[21] makes a case that abuse of caffeine-containing powders for their mood altering effects has an important influence on the occurrence of analgesic nephropathy. He found that most analgesic tablets are usually taken in moderate amounts for appropriate indications for the relief of pain whereas caffeine-containing powders are used in excessive quantities for their mood altering properties. In almost all countries in which analgesic nephropathy is a serious problem, caffeine-containing analgesic powders are the major culprit.

Data from Australia tend to support Murray's[21] view in that 55% of mixed analgesic powder sales (containing caffeine) were made through food stores and only 5% through pharmacies, whereas 54% of tablets were sold through pharmacies[22]. It seems likely that pharmacists are more likely to be consulted when the patient is seeking pain relief, whereas powders were regarded as part of the weekly grocery order. Analgesic powders were sold by supermarkets in packets containing one gross.

TABLE 1.2 End-stage renal failure due to analgesic nephropathy and analgesic consumption in Australia

State	*Proportion of population taking analgesics daily (%)*		*No. of patients with papillary necrosis entering dialysis transplantation programme per year per million population*	*No. of patients entering programme with analgesic nephropathy (%)*
	Females	*Males*		
Victoria	5	3	1.3	5.2
Western Australia	3	3	2.3	—
South Australia	—	—	4.3	16.8
Queensland	16	11	6.7	29
New South Wales	9	5	8.4	27

(Reproduced from Ref. 140)

Scotland shows a very high prevalence of analgesic nephropathy in West Glasgow where a particular powder containing aspirin, phenacetin and caffeine is widely advertised[21]. In Belgium, analgesic abuse is frequent in an area of Antwerp adjacent to three factories which manufacture mixed analgesic powders[23,24].

In Australia, the frequency of analgesic nephropathy appears to be higher in those states where a larger percentage of the population takes analgesics daily (Table 1.2). Analgesic sales in one country town in Queensland were at the rate of 1.8 g phenacetin per head of the population per year[25].

Relatively few formal studies have been carried out to assess the frequency of analgesic intake in the community. Waters *et al.*[26] surveyed women aged 20–64 years living in a Welsh industrial valley;

1.9% took more than four analgesic tablets daily but this percentage was as high as 3.7% in women aged 45–54.

In Newcastle, New South Wales, which has the highest prevalence of renal papillary necrosis in Australia, 5.4% of women and 3.7% of men take analgesics daily. These findings are surprisingly close to the reports from Waters[26] in spite of the low prevalence of analgesic nephropathy in the United Kingdom. Purnell and Burry[25] found that 12% of the population of a country town in Queensland took analgesics daily, whereas we found that only 2.6% of the population in a coastal resort in Victoria took 2000 mg of aspirin (that is 4–5 tablets) per week.

Whereas, in Australia, these studies documenting analgesic intake in the community appear to correlate with the frequency of analgesic nephropathy, the rarity of papillary necrosis at autopsy in the United Kingdom (Table 1.1) is difficult to explain – especially since Waters[26] found that a relatively high percentage of women take 4–5 analgesic tablets daily.

The different pattern of analgesic consumption in Australia is reflected in differences in the numbers of patients presenting with end-stage renal failure due to analgesic nephropathy in the different States (Table 1.2). The increasing prevalence of renal papillary necrosis shown in various countries during the 1950–1970s period (Table 1.1) is likely to be declining in most countries at this time. Figure 1.1 shows the declining proportion of patients with analgesic nephropathy among those presenting for dialysis in Australia. Even more striking than this figure is the disappearance of patients with analgesic nephropathy from the clinics and the wards[27, 28]. New patients with analgesic nephropathy have become curiosities and the lecture on this topic has been dropped from our undergraduate curriculum in Melbourne.

The most important epidemiological study which establishes that heavy analgesic abuse causes renal damage is that of Dubach and his colleagues[29]. This prospective longitudinal study compared 623 women in Switzerland who had objective evidence of analgesic consumption with 621 women who did not. These women were followed for 11 years. At the beginning of the study, the women who took analgesics had a higher mean serum creatinine concentration and lower mean specific gravity of urine than the control group. At the end of the 11-year period, overall mortality, mortality due to renal disease and mortality due to cardiovascular disease were all higher in the women taking analgesics.

Clinical aspects

Analgesic nephropathy

Analgesic nephropathy occurs predominantly in middle-aged women who take analgesics for inappropriate reasons – usually for mood-altering effects[30]. The renal manifestations are part of a clinical syndrome which involves other systems. Almost all patients show evidence of personality disorders or neurosis and one third of our patients[31] and half of Murray's patients[30] had undergone previous psychiatric treatment. The underlying psychiatric abnormalities have been regarded by most as the reason why patients take excessive quantities of analgesics. It has also been suggested that analgesics may cause dementia[32].

Gastrointestinal abnormalities occur in a third to a half of all patients with analgesic nephropathy[31,33] and frank peptic ulceration in a third of patients. Anaemia, a common manifestation in early studies[31], may be due to haemolysis, gastrointestinal blood loss or chronic renal failure[33].

Atheroma seems to be inappropriately severe in relation to the age of the patients and ischaemic heart disease was a prominent cause of mortality in our original series of patients, accounting for 25% of deaths[31]. Some women died in their 30s of ischaemic heart disease. Atheromatous lesions in other large vessels were also prominent, including peripheral vascular disease and renal artery stenosis. Atheromatous renal artery stenosis is usually rare in women under the age of 50 years and was significantly increased in women with analgesic nephropathy[34]. Nanra's group have reported ischaemic heart disease in 33% of patients with analgesic nephropathy[35].

Hypertension is frequently present and may be more common in patients with the analgesic syndrome in Australia than in Europe. Sixty percent of patients in Australian series are hypertensive compared with 15–40% in some European studies. Over 80% of uraemic patients are hypertensive[36]. Malignant hypertension may occur and patients may develop this complication in spite of marked sodium depletion. The

TABLE 1.3 Functional changes in analgesic nephropathy

	Incidence (%)
Impaired concentration capacity	100
Sterile pyuria	50–100
Renal insufficiency	78.8
Hypertension	
Benign	15–70
Malignant	6.1
Urinary tract infection	15–69
Proteinuria	38.5
Haematuria	33.5
Urinary acidification	
Impaired	25.3
Renal tubular acidosis	9.3
Clinical gout	21.1
Salt depletion	—
Septicaemia	—

(Reproduced from Ref. 37)
— = data not available

possibility of an underlying renal artery stenosis should be considered especially in severe cases. Repair of renal artery stenosis may result in better control of hypertension and improved renal function.

Renal manifestations

Renal manifestations are listed in Tables 1.3 and 1.4[37].

In the acute stage, patients typically have sterile pyuria, macroscopic or microscopic haematuria, episodes of impaired renal function which frequently recover with appropriate management and episodes of renal colic due to passing of separated papillae down the ureter. Sterile pyuria is a good marker of activity of the papillary necrosis and, while it persists, the patient is probably continuing to take analgesics and show active renal lesions.

An unequivocal diagnosis of renal papillary necrosis depends upon demonstration of characteristic medullary or papillary cavities on radiographs or upon the histological demonstration of necrotic papillae tissue in the urine. Another less frequent but diagnostic radiological feature is the demonstration of calcification around the rim of a separated papilla.

TABLE 1.4 Morphological changes in analgesic nephropathy

	Incidence (%)
Renal papillary necrosis	100
Glomerular lesions[a]	69.9
Medullary calcification	35.9
Renal calculi	—
Transitional cell carcinoma	—
Hydronephrosis/pyonephrosis	—
Ureteric stricture	—
Atheromatous renal artery stenosis	—
Renal vein thrombosis	—
Interstitial cystitis	—

[a]In patients with proteinuria
— = data not available
(Reproduced from Ref. 37)

Uroepithelial carcinoma
In 1965, Hultengren and Lagergren[38] described 11 cases of renal carcinoma in 103 cases of renal papillary necrosis. Subsequent reports have come from other groups[39–41]. There is now no doubt that patients with analgesic nephropathy have an increased risk of uroepithelial tumours in the bladder or renal pelvis.

Investigations

Urine microscopy:
Sterile pyuria is an important finding during the active phase of renal papillary necrosis. In addition, most patients have episodes of urinary tract infection. These are usually renal infections and, if obstruction is present, may lead to septicaemia and death[31].

During episodes of macroscopic haematuria which occur in relation to separation of papillae, urinary erythrocyte counts exceed 5×10^6. Morphologically, erythrocytes are always non-glomerular. Macroscopic haematuria may be present while active disease persists but disappears when analgesic abuse ceases – as does the sterile pyuria. Later reappearance of microscopic haematuria indicates one of two complications. If glomerular microscopic haematuria recurs, then a secondary, progressive glomerular lesion will be found on biopsy – typically focal and segmental hyalinosis and sclerosis. If non-glomerular haematuria is present, a uroepithelial malignancy may have developed.

Urine protein:
Even with severe impairment of renal function, urine protein levels may be within the normal range (<0.2 g/24h) but commonly increases to 0.2–0.5 g in 24 hours. When a secondary glomerular lesion develops, much higher urine protein levels may occur and occasionally these patients develop nephrotic syndrome.

Papillary fragments:
In a case of suspected active renal papillary necrosis, the urine should be strained for renal papillary tissue which is often brown or black in colour macroscopically and shows necrotic papillary tissue microscopically. If a calculus is passed, it should be decalcified and sectioned and may contain necrotic papillary tissue.

Renal function tests:
Serum urea and creatinine concentrations may be raised but, even where they are normal, the creatinine clearance and urine concentrating capacity are often abnormal. Urinary acidification is also usually impaired.

Bladder biopsy:
The characteristic appearance of small blood vessels in the bladder mucosa has also been occasionally used to diagnose analgesic nephropathy[20].

Radiological investigations:
The radiological features of renal papillary necrosis may be diagnostic. A diagrammatic representation of papillary and medullary cavities and other characteristic lesions is shown in Figure 1.4.

In the early stages of the disease, renal size may be normal even when there are papillary cavities or separated papillae in papillary

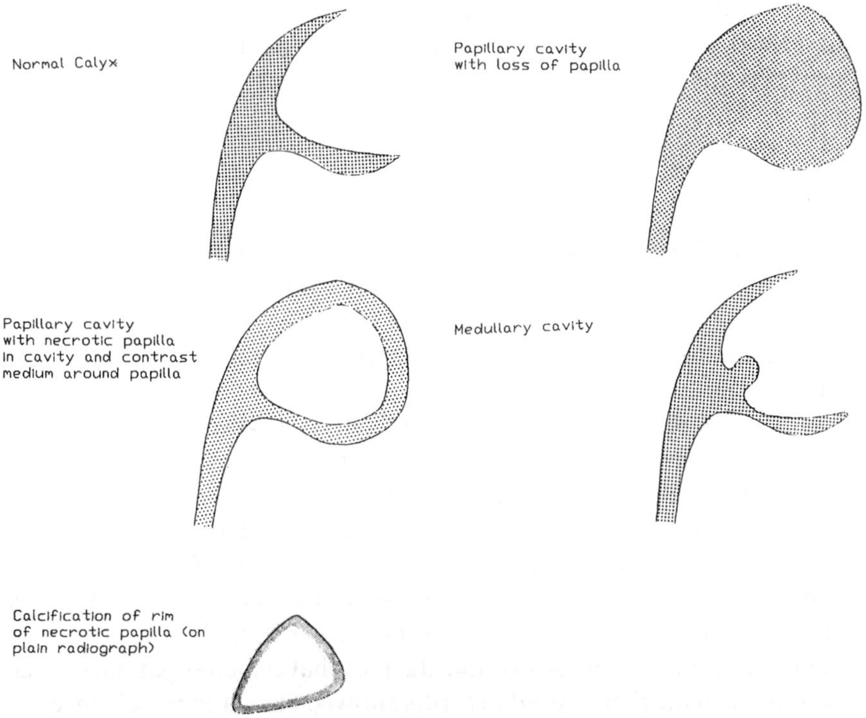

FIGURE 1.4 Diagrammatic representation of characteristic calyceal changes seen radiographically in renal papillary necrosis

cavities as evidence of papillary necrosis. Rapid reduction in renal size may occur following an episode of papillary separation. The changes are usually bilateral and affect all papillae. It has recently been shown that there may be no positive radiological findings in calices where all papillae remain attached to the so-called *in situ* lesion[16]. A normal intravenous pyelogram does not exclude a diagnosis of renal papillary necrosis.

Ureteric stricture and retroperitoneal fibrosis have been documented in several cases[42–44]. Retrograde or antigrade pyelography may be necessary if the ureter is obstructed by papillary tissue or to exclude or establish a diagnosis of uroepithelial neoplasm. Renal angiography may be indicated if renal artery stenosis is suspected.

Newer imaging techniques such as CAT scanning, may be useful in detecting early uroepithelial neoplasms. Ultrasonic features have been described in patients with end-stage renal failure due to analgesic nephropathy[45]. Essentially this method reveals calcified renal papillae.

Renal papillary necrosis associated with NSAIDs

Renal papillary necrosis has been associated with NSAIDs in rheumatoid arthritis, juvenile rheumatoid arthritis and ankylosing spondylitis[46].

Several autopsy studies of renal papillary necrosis in patients with rheumatoid arthritis have revealed macroscopic evidence of renal papillary necrosis in 7–26% of cases (Table 1.5). Microscopic evidence was present in 57% of cases in our controlled study of all autopsy kidneys over a 12-month period. Eight percent of 641 autopsy kidneys at the Royal Melbourne Hospital showed renal papillary necrosis compared with 2.8% of 538 kidneys examined at the Coroner's court over the same period[47]. The 57% incidence of renal papillary necrosis in cases with rheumatoid arthritis is particularly significant in view of the blind nature of the study and the fact that hospital patients other than those with rheumatoid arthritis showed such a low incidence.

Renal papillary necrosis has been described in three patients with juvenile rheumatoid arthritis in whom the major treatment was high-dose, long-term aspirin[48]. This is the clinical counterpart to experimental studies which demonstrated papillary necrosis in rats receiving aspirin and is of significance in relation to the view that aspirin may be an important factor in analgesic nephropathy[4]. One of these patients had ingested ibuprofen and tolmetin for short periods, one had taken tolmetin for a year and paracetamol for a brief period, and the third aspirin alone. We reported two cases in both of whom indomethacin had been used long term with short-term intermittent aspirin or paracetamol[49].

In adults with rheumatoid arthritis, the chronic nature of the disease and complex therapeutic protocols make it difficult to determine the specific cause of the papillary necrosis. The drugs taken by 20 patients with renal papillary necrosis and rheumatoid arthritis whom we reported are shown in Table 1.6.

Renal papillary necrosis in man has been attributed to phenyl-

TABLE 1.5 Autopsy incidence of renal papillary necrosis and chronic interstitial nephritis in rheumatoid arthritis

Rheumatoid arthritis studies	*Incidence at autopsy*		
	Renal papillary necrosis		*Chronic Interstitial Nephritis*
	Macroscopic evidence	*Microscopic evidence*	
Clausen and Pedersen, 1961	18/80 (22.5%)	—	—
Lawson and McLean, 1966	13/61 (21.3%)	18/61 (29.5%)	29/61 (47.5%)
Gardner, 1969	11/142 (7.8%)	—	—
Burry *et al.*, 1974	—	4/22 (18.2%)	—
Present study	6/23 (26.1%)	12/21 (57.1%)	12/23 (52.2%)

(Reproduced from Ref. 141)

TABLE 1.6 Medications taken by 20 patients with rheumatoid arthritis

	No. of patients
Aspirin	20
Prednisolone	11
Codeine phosphate	8
Phenylbutazone	7
Paracetamol	5
Indomethacin	5
APC mixture	4
Chloroquin	4
Gold	3
Mefenamic acid	2
Propoxyphene HCl	1

(Reproduced from Ref. 142).

butazone[50–52], indomethacin[53], naproxen and benoxaprofen[54,55]. In animals, almost all NSAIDs have produced renal papillary necrosis and it is likely that individual reports of cases with renal papillary necrosis in man will continue to appear as newer NSAIDs are introduced.

The clinical features of renal papillary necrosis seen with NSAIDs are similar to, but less severe than those in analgesic nephropathy. This may be related to the fact that the papillae tend to remain attached or *in situ* in the patients taking only aspirin or NSAIDs. Because of this, the complications which occur during separation of papillae, such as haematuria, ureteric obstruction, severe urinary tract infection, and septicaemia are not usually seen. Hypertension has also been infrequent in the small number of patients reported and psychiatric manifestations are absent.

There is no evidence of an increased risk of either atheromatous complications or uroepithelial carcinoma in patients with renal papillary necrosis due to NSAIDs. The overall risk of developing impaired renal function appears to be small in patients with rheumatoid arthritis[56] in spite of the high incidence of renal papillary necrosis at autopsy (Table 1.5).

Course and management of renal papillary necrosis

Although end-stage renal failure occurs if renal papillary necrosis due to analgesics or NSAIDs progresses, considerable recovery of renal function may occur if the patients stop ingesting all analgesics and NSAIDs[36]. Such patients do not usually die of renal failure which remains stable for many years; other complications of the analgesic syndrome, such as myocardial infarction, are the usual cause of death.

When phenacetin was thought to be the sole cause of analgesic nephropathy, many companies removed phenacetin from compound preparations and substituted paracetamol or salicylate. In our experience[36] and that of other groups[57,58], renal function continues to decline unless ingestion of all over-the-counter analgesics, including aspirin, ceases; the chances of recovery of renal function are then excellent (Figure 1.5) and maintained long term. Some of our patients who presented in 1959 with impaired renal function died 15–20 years later

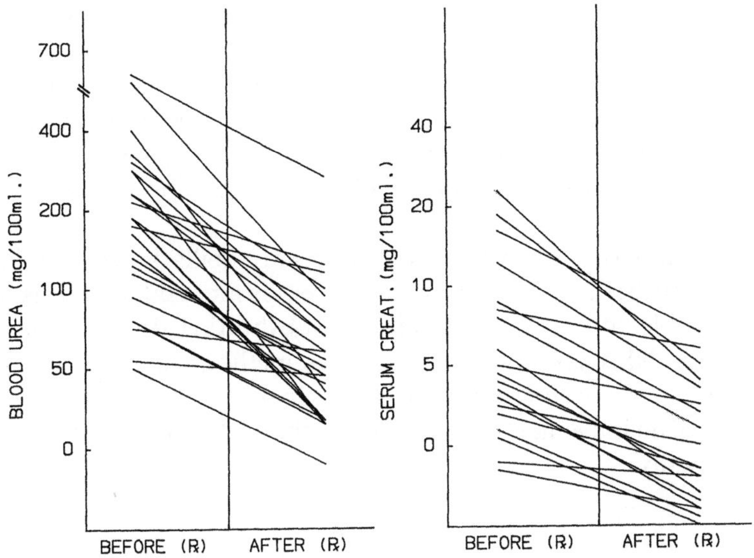

FIGURE 1.5 Improvement in blood urea and serum creatinine concentrations after treatment in patients with analgesic nephropathy and impaired renal function. (From Ref. 36)

without showing any subsequent deterioration in function.

Apart from withdrawal of the offending drugs, other factors are important in ensuring recovery of renal function in analgesic nephropathy.

Diagnosis and relief of ureteric obstruction which is extremely common during episodes of papillary separation, are clearly important. Treatment of infection is also important, even if ureteric obstruction is not present. The nature of the lesion of renal papillary necrosis creates intrarenal obstruction. This in turn causes lesions within the renal parenchyma in the affected nephrons and this 'infected obstructed' area may be associated with severe symptoms and even septicaemia. There is intrarenal obstruction by necrotic papillae. Renal infection may, thereby, not only contribute to impairment of renal function but may be complicated by episodes of septicaemia.

Patients with analgesic nephropathy are often severely salt and water depleted; for optimum recovery these abnormalities must be corrected.

Hypertension is often severe, even malignant, and may be refractory to treatment. Sometimes dehydration and correction of sodium depletion improve blood pressure control. In these patients, no attempt should be made to control hypertension by further sodium depletion.

In patients with arthritis who have renal papillary necrosis due to aspirin or other NSAIDs, the management is more difficult. It is often not possible to control the pain by substituting drugs other than aspirin or NSAIDs but drugs, such as methotrexate, penicillamine and steroids, have been used successfully in some of our patients. Other aspects of management are similar to those described for analgesic nephropathy.

Which drug or drug combination is responsible for renal papillary necrosis?

Many drugs may thus cause renal papillary necrosis. It now seems extraordinary that analgesic nephropathy was so readily attributed only to phenacetin in the early studies. This conclusion was based purely on the fact that phenacetin was an ingredient of most of the drug combinations taken by patients with analgesic nephropathy. It would be just as logical to blame caffeine which is also a component of almost all the over-the-counter medications concerned. The obvious illogicality of this reasoning was pointed out by Gilman in 1964[59]. 'If scotch and soda, brandy and soda and vodka and soda all cause inebriation, then soda is clearly responsible for this effect.'

It is now quite clear that almost all NSAIDs cause renal papillary necrosis in experimental animals. We have produced papillary necrosis using phenylbutazone, mefenamic acid, indomethacin, phenazone and propoxyphene[60,61]. Others have produced papillary necrosis with sudoxicam[62], aminopyrine, phenazone, antipyrine[63], fenamic acids[64] and fenoprofen[53].

These experimental studies are relevant to the small number of patients who develop papillary necrosis while taking pharmacological doses of NSAIDs. One recent experimental finding is particularly relevant to this group of patients. We have found that caffeine greatly increases the incidence of papillary necrosis in rats receiving NSAIDs[65]. This may mean that patients with arthritis on NSAIDs should not drink excessive quantities of tea and coffee. As NSAIDs, sometimes in combination with caffeine, are now available without a prescription over the counter in several countries, it may also warrant a warning on packages.

These observations on NSAIDs are relevant to analgesic nephropathy which results from excessive use of over-the-counter analgesics. Aspirin, like other NSAIDs, produces renal papillary necrosis in rats[66] and there is mounting evidence that it also does so in man[53]. Phenacetin, on the other hand produces no papillary changes unless it is given to rats in heroic doses and it never produces the florid lesions seen with NSAIDs, aspirin and with mixed analgesics[60,61]. In man, there is overwhelming evidence that a variety of combinations of aspirin, phenacetin, phenazone, salicylamide, paracetamol and caffeine can produce renal papillary necrosis.

Control measures which sought to remove only phenacetin worked in those countries in which phenacetin was combined with non-aspirin containing medications. In Australia, the epidemic of analgesic nephropathy continued unabated in spite of removal of phenacetin from many over-the-counter preparations in 1962 and from all but one in 1967. In 1975 the last phenacetin was withdrawn from over-the-counter drugs but no discernible reduction in the prevalence of analgesic nephropathy occurred over this 13-year period during which phenacetin sales fell from very high levels to zero. Because of this and because patients did not improve when phenacetin was no longer ingested but other drugs, such as paracetamol, aspirin and salicylamide, were continued, restrictions were introduced in Australia to prevent over-the-counter sales of:

(1) Mixtures of any two analgesics;
(2) Mixtures containing caffeine;
(3) Packs containing more than 25 tablets.

Following such legislation in 1980, there has been a dramatic reduction in the number of clinical cases of analgesic nephropathy and there is a steady decline each year in the percentage of patients with analgesic nephropathy requiring dialysis (Figure 1.1). This has occurred in spite of an increase of the age of patients accepted for dialysis; this is relevant because analgesic nephropathy causes end-stage renal failure mainly in women over the age of 60.

Although Canada initially reported a declining incidence of analgesic nephropathy following withdrawal of phenacetin, this improvement was not sustained[67]. The NIM Consensus panel, which met in 1984, recommended withdrawal of mixed analgesic drugs from over-the-counter use. They recommended that, as in Australia, only single antipyretic analgesics should be available over-the-counter[68].

Causative mechanisms

The mechanisms producing renal papillary necrosis in analgesic nephropathy are controversial; a direct toxic effect and/or an ischaemic process may be involved. The increasing emphasis on NSAIDs as a cause of renal papillary necrosis lends support to the view that a reduction in medullary blood flow due to inhibition of vasodilatory prostaglandins may be an important factor in renal papillary necrosis.

Discussion

Hopefully analgesic nephropathy will soon be relegated to the history of medicine. Its explosive appearance in the middle of this century reached a peak in Australia where it was found at autopsy in 20% of cases (Table 1.5) and was the cause of end-stage renal failure in 25% of cases presenting for dialysis – even when the upper age limit for dialysis acceptance was about 60 years. Clinical cases of this condition are now rare and the percentage of patients with this disease requiring dialysis has fallen to 11%, most of whom are elderly women (Figure 1.1).

Analgesic nephropathy still accounts for substantial numbers of patients entering dialysis programmes in some European countries, notably Belgium and Switzerland. The rate of acceptance does not

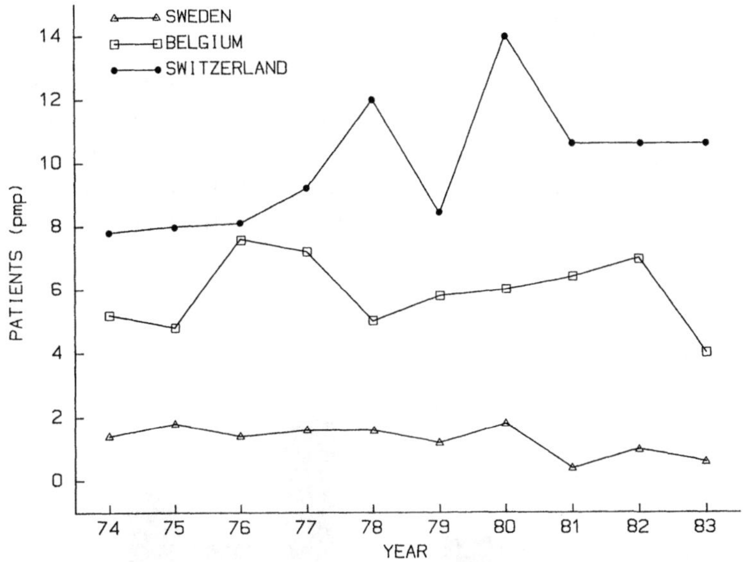

FIGURE 1.6 Age-specific acceptance rates for dialysis for patients aged less than 65 years with end-stage renal failure due to analgesic nephropathy, 1974–83 in Switzerland, Belgium and Sweden

appear to be falling (Figure 1.6). The high rate of acceptance of patients with analgesic nephropathy in Belgium contrasts with a much lower acceptance rate in other countries, such as the United Kingdom and France. Age-specific acceptance rates for women in Belgium and France show very large differences (Figure 1.7). The continuing problem of analgesic nephropathy in countries such as Belgium and Switzerland is due to continued high uncontrolled sales of over-the-counter mixed analgesic compounds.

A disturbing factor is the recent appearance of analgesic nephropathy in third world countries. As in the tobacco industry, when restrictions are introduced and sales fall in the developing world, the multinational companies selling mixed analgesics now concentrate their advertising and sales in third world countries. Reports are now appearing of significant numbers of cases of analgesic nephropathy from countries such as Malaysia[69–75].

ACUTE EFFECTS OF NSAIDs ON THE KIDNEY

The first reports of acute nephrotoxic effects of NSAIDs were probably our own. We reported a severe deterioration in renal function in individual patients with analgesic nephropathy who, having ceased all analgesic medication, started to take aspirin, either alone or in combination with paracetamol, which they or their doctors believed

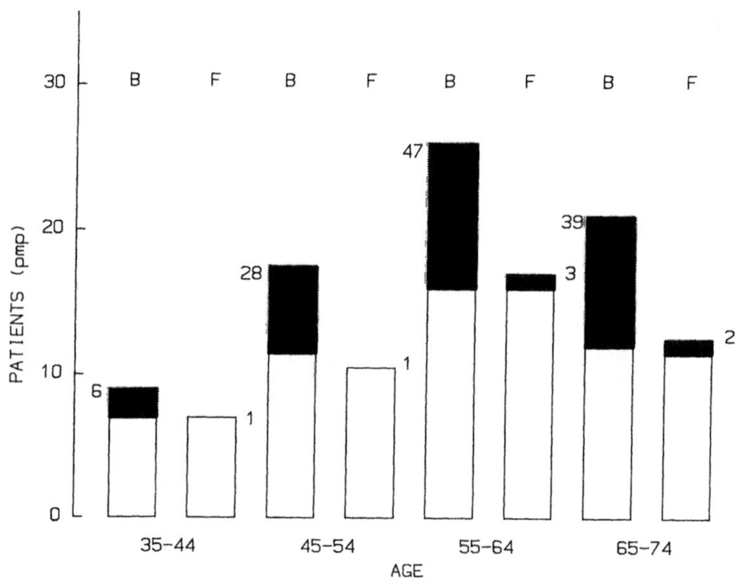

FIGURE 1.7 Age-specific acceptance rates per million population for renal replacement therapy in women commencing treatment 1981–83 in Belgium (B) and France (F). Acceptance rates for those with analgesic nephropathy are shown as shaded area

to be safe[36,60]. Michielsen *et al.* in 1973 reported a sudden decline in the GFR of patients with glomerulonephritis given indomethacin[76]. In 1977 Kimberley and Plotz reported a reduction in creatinine clearance when aspirin was given to patients with lupus nephritis[77]. It is now well recognized that NSAIDs often cause an acute deterioration in renal function when given to patients with impaired renal function[78–83].

This decline in renal function is attributed to the greater dependence of patients with renal disease on secretion of PGE_2 and prostacyclin for the maintenance of renal blood flow. Prostaglandins are said to maintain blood flow by efferent arteriolar dilatation; NSAIDs inhibit production of PGE_2 and PGI_2 and thus produce an acute reduction in renal blood flow. Sulindac, which is a selective inhibitor of extra-renal cyclo-oxygenase, is said to be less likely to cause impairment of renal function in patients with renal disease[84,85].

If deterioration were due solely to a change in renal blood flow in patients with renal disease, it should, in theory, be reversible as soon as the drug is stopped. In 1970, however, we reported[36] a permanent deterioration in renal function and fresh episodes of renal papillary necrosis in some patients with renal disease given aspirin or aspirin combinations. In most cases, a prompt improvement in renal function follows withdrawal of the NSAID, but acute tubular necrosis has rarely been demonstrated on biopsy[86].

In high renin states induced by sodium depletion[87], heart failure[88] or cirrhosis[89,90], NSAIDs may also cause an acute deterioration in renal function. A similar effect has been described in patients given a NSAID and diuretics. Many such patients were receiving triamterene and other mechanisms, such as crystal obstruction of the tubules, may perhaps be relevant[91].

Hyperkalaemia

Severe hyperkalaemia may accompany an acute decline in renal function[81]. This has been noted particularly when indomethacin was used to treat gout in patients with impaired renal function[82]. It has also been reported, however, in patients with normal renal function[92] while severe hyperkalaemia, out of proportion to the degree of impairment, has been recorded in those with decreased renal function[93–96].

All NSAIDs, with the possible exception of sulindac[84], reduce plasma renin activity and suppress aldosterone secretion. Resulting hyporeninaemic hypoaldosteronism has been invoked as the cause of hyperkalaemia[82] which also occurs in infants given indomethacin therapy for patent ductus arteriosus[97].

Acute renal failure and nephrotic syndrome associated with acute interstitial nephritis

Patients receiving non-steroidal anti-inflammatory drugs may develop severe acute renal failure requiring dialysis. Within this group there are two distinct clinical syndromes occurring under different circumstances and with different pathological findings and prognosis. Distinction between the two is important and only occasionally difficult.

Acute renal failure

Acute renal failure, even when severe, may be prerenal and due to the haemodynamic factors discussed above. Many of the patients who develop the syndrome of acute renal failure will show underlying acute tubular necrosis; recovery is delayed 10–14 days and dialysis may be necessary.

This syndrome is seen in the same group of patients who develop a temporary deterioration in renal function when given NSAIDs and may represent a more severe extension of the same process. Patients with high renin states, advanced age, concurrent use of diuretics and underlying renal vascular disease are most susceptible[98]. It has also been documented in patients with congestive cardiac failure, cirrhosis with ascites, infants with patent ductus arteriosus and in the nephrotic syndrome[79,88,89].

Although some of these patients recover promptly, suggesting that haemodynamic factors account for the deterioration in renal function[99], acute tubular necrosis has been documented histologically in others[100]. Patients with acute gout seem to be particularly liable to develop this form of acute renal failure[98].

Indomethacin has been the drug responsible in most reported cases of this syndrome of acute renal failure but it has also been the most widely prescribed NSAID over many years. The earliest records of acute renal failure with NSAIDs occurred in patients with gout receiving phenylbutazone[101–103]. Phenylbutazone, unlike most other NSAIDs, is a powerful uricosuric agent and it is possible that acute renal failure with phenylbutazone is due to a different mechanism which involves uric acid crystal deposition in tubules. Sulphinpyrazone, which is a derivative of phenylbutazone but not a NSAID, also causes acute renal failure[104–108]. The relationship between deposits of uric acid crystals in tubules and acute renal failure with these two uricosuric agents remains unresolved. It is noteworthy, however, that tienelic acid, another uricosuric agent also causes acute renal failure[109–111]. It may well be that uric acid crystal deposition is one factor in the acute renal failure documented in patients receiving phenylbutazone.

Mefenamic acid has been implicated in many patients as a cause of NSAID-associated renal failure leading to the name 'mefenamic acid nephropathy'[112]. Unfortunately, the cases described under this title had a variety of clinico-pathological associations; one had interstitial nephritis[113]; one had an associated generalized vasculitis[114]; and one occurred in a patient receiving triamterene and mefenamic acid, and, as discussed above, crystalluria due to triamterene may have been a contributing factor[91].

Overall data suggest that the major mechanisms involved in the syndrome of acute renal failure in patients receiving NSAIDs are haemodynamic. In milder cases, the acute deterioration may be prerenal and prompt recovery follows withdrawal of NSAIDs; in others, acute tubular necrosis develops but it is likely that the mechanism which causes acute tubular necrosis is ischaemic and not toxic[80,81,100,115–119].

Acute interstitial nephritis and the nephrotic syndrome

This syndrome includes a wide spectrum of cases ranging from the nephrotic syndrome without clear-cut acute interstitial nephritis on biopsy at one end[120] to acute interstitial nephritis without the nephrotic syndrome at the other[113,120–124].

There are several points which distinguish this clinical syndrome from the cases of acute renal failure due to haemodynamic factors discussed above. This syndrome appears to be idiosyncratic and certain drugs are particularly likely to be involved. Fenoprofen accounts for two-thirds of the reported cases and other relatively infrequently used drugs, such as zomepirac and tolmetin, have been implicated as the cause in five and four cases respectively. Single case reports have appeared in patients receiving a range of drugs, including mefenamic acid, ibuprofen, naproxen and indomethacin[113,120–137]. We have recently recorded four cases in patients receiving sulindac.

The clinical context in which this syndrome occurs is different. It does not occur more frequently in patients with predisposing factors, such as old age, underlying renal disease or high renin states. The onset has been documented between 2 months and 18 months of the start of NSAID treatment whereas the acute renal failure syndrome due to haemodynamic factors often comes on within days of the first dose. Unlike other drug-related causes of acute interstitial nephritis, the patients do not have a rash, fever or eosinophilia and there is no eosinophiluria.

The nephrotic syndrome may be severe and renal failure usually requires dialysis. Unlike the syndrome of acute renal failure, recovery does not occur when the NSAID is withdrawn. In many patients, renal function remains permanently impaired and the nephrotic syndrome may persist for months.

While the place of steroid therapy is unresolved, prompt resolution of the nephrotic syndrome and recovery of renal function may occur when steroid treatment is given. This may occur even when both impaired renal function and the nephrotic syndrome have been present and unaltered for some weeks. A trial of a short course of steroids is therefore recommended.

Clive and Stoff[138] have calculated that one in seven persons in the United States is taking a NSAID. It is not surprising, therefore, that these clinical syndromes are two of the most frequent drug-related causes of acute renal failure and the nephrotic syndrome presenting to renal units at this time.

REFERENCES

1. Spuhler, O. and Zollinger, H.U. (1953). Die chronisch-interstitielle Nephritis. *Zeitschrift Klinische Medizin*, **151**, 1–50
2. Nanra, R.S. and Kincaid-Smith, P. (1972). Chronic effect of analgesics on the kidney. In Edwards, K.D.G. (ed.) *Drugs Affecting Kidney Function and Metabolism. Progress in Biochemical Pharmacology*, Chap. 7, pp. 285–323. (Basel: Karger)
3. Adams, D.H., Howie, A.J., Michael, J., Bacon, P.A., McConkey, B. and Adu,

D. (1986). Non-steroidal anti-inflammatory drugs and renal failure. *Lancet*, **2,** 57–59
4. Nanra, R. S. and Kincaid-Smith, P. (1973). Experimental and clinical analgesic nephropathy with aspirin. In Haschek, H. (ed.) *Phenacetin Abuse 1973. International Symposium on Problems of Phenacetin Abuse, Vienna 1973*, pp. 89–114. (Vienna: Facta Publications)
5. Schourup, K. (1957). Necrosis of the renal papillae. Post-mortem series. *Acta Pathol. Microbiol. Scand.*, **41,** 462–478
6. Lindeneg, O., Fisher, S., Pedersen, J. and Nissen, N.I. (1959). Necrosis of the renal papillae and prolonged abuse of phenacetin. *Acta Med. Scand.*, **165,** 321–328
7. Davson, J. and Langley, F. A. (1944). Papillitis renis necroticans. *J. Pathol. Bact.*, **56,** 327
8. Knutsen, A., Jennings, E. R., Osborne, A., Brines, O. A. and Axelrod, A. (1952). Renal papillary necrosis. *Am. J. Clin. Pathol.*, **22,** 327–336
9. Kincaid-Smith, P. (1967). Pathogenesis of the renal lesion associated with the abuse of analgesics. *Lancet*, **1,** 850–862
10. Kincaid-Smith, P. (1963). The association between chronic renal disease, peptic ulceration and analgesic abuse. *Proceedings of the 2nd International Congress of Nephrology, Prague. Excerpta Medica International Congress Series*, **67,** 91
11. Kincaid-Smith, P. (1965). Bacteriuria in pregnancy. In Kass, E. H. (ed.) *Progress in Pyelonephritis*, pp. 360. (Philadelphia: Davis)
12. Saker, B. M. and Kincaid-Smith, P. (1969). Papillary necrosis in experimental analgesic nephropathy. *Brit. Med. J.*, **1,** 161–162
13. Davies, D. J. (1968). Changes in the renal cortex following experimental medullary necrosis. *Arch. Pathol.*, **86,** 377–382
14. Lucke, V. M., Messery, M., Lucke, J. N. and Hunt, A. C. (1968). Effects on the kidney of removal of the renal papilla. *Arch. Pathol.*, **86,** 390–394
15. Burry, A. F. (1967). The evolution of analgesic nephropathy.*Nephron*, **5,** 185–201
16. Fairley, K. F. and Kincaid-Smith, P. (1968). Renal papillary necrosis with a normal pyelogram. *Brit. Med. J.*, **1,** 156–157
17. Burry, A. F. (1978). Pathology of analgesic nephropathy: Australian experience. *Kidney Int.*, **13,** 34–40
18. Gloor, F. J. (1978). Changing concepts in pathogenesis and morphology of analgesic nephropathy as seen in Europe. *Kidney Int.*, **13,** 27–33
19. Kincaid-Smith, P., Saker, B. M., McKenzie, I. F. C. and Muirden, K. C. (1968). Lesions in the blood supply of the papilla in experimental analgesic nephropathy. *Med. J. Aust.*, **1,** 203–206
20. Izak, J. V., Fourie, H., Pauw, F. H. and de Bruin, B. (1982). Bladder urothelium in analgesic-associated nephropathy – A valuable diagnostic aid. *J. Urol*, **128,** 262–263
21. Murray, R. M. (1978). Genesis of analgesic nephropathy in the United Kingdom. *Kidney Int.*, **13,** 50–57
22. The Senate Standing Committee on Social Welfare (1977). *Drug problems in Australia – an intoxicated society?* (Canberra: Government Publ. Service)
23. Michielson, P., de Schepper, P. J., de Broe, M., Valkenborgh, G. and Tricot, J. P. (1972). Renal disease due to drugs. In Meyler, L. and Peck, H. M. (eds.) *Drug Induced Diseases*, Chap. 4, pp. 261–314. (Amsterdam: Excerpta Medica)

24. Vanderweghem, J. L. and Even-Adin, D. (1982). Epidemiology of analgesic nephropathy in Belgium. *Clin. Nephrol.*, **17,** 129–133
25. Purnell, J. and Burry, A. F. (1967). Analgesic consumption in a country town. *Med. J. Aust.*, **2,** 389–391
26. Waters, W. E., Elwood, P. C. and Asscher, W. W. (1973). Community survey of analgesic consumption and kidney function in women. *Lancet*, **1,** 341–344
27. Egger, G., O'Neill, P., Nanra, R. S. and Leeder, S. R. (1979). Prevalence of compound analgesic use in Newcastle (NSW). *Aust. Family Physician*, **8,** 777–782
28. Christie, D., McPherson, L. and Kincaid-Smith, P. (1976). Analgesics and the kidney – a community-based study. *Med. J. Aust.*, **2,** 527–529
29. Dubach, U. C., Rosner, B. and Pfister, E. (1983). Epidemiologic study of abuse of analgesics containing phenacetin. *N. Engl. J. Med.*, **308,** 357–362
30. Murray, R. M. (1973). The origins of analgesic nephropathy. *Brit. J. Psychiat.*, **123,** 99–106
31. Dawborn, J. K., Fairley, K. F., Kincaid-Smith, P. and King, W. E. (1966). The association of peptic ulceration, chronic renal disease and analgesic abuse. *Q.J. Med.*, **35,** (137(4)), 69–83
32. Murray, R. M., Greene, J. G. and Adams, J. H. (1971). Analgesic abuse and dementia. *Lancet*, **2,** 242–246
33. Nanra, R. S. (1976). Analgesic nephropathy. *Med. J. Aust.*, **1,** 745
34. Kincaid-Smith, P. (1979). Analgesic nephropathy in Australia. In Kuhn, K. and Brod, J. (eds.) *Contributions to Nephrology: Interstitial Nephropathies, 6th Symposium on Nephrology*, Hanover, May 1978, 16, 57–64. (Basel/Hanover: Karger)
35. Krishnaswamy, S., Wallace, D. C. and Nanra, R. S. (1974). Ischaemic heart disease in analgesic nephropathy. *Aust. N.Z. J. Med.*, **4,** 426
36. Kincaid-Smith, P., Nanra, R. S. and Fairley, K. F. (1971). Analgesic nephropathy: a recoverable form of chronic renal failure. In Kincaid-Smith, P. and Fairley, K. F. (eds.) *Renal Infection and Renal Scarring*, pp. 385–400. (Melbourne: Mercedes Publishing Services)
37. Kincaid-Smith, P. and Nanra, R. S. (1979). Renal medullary necrosis. In Hamburger, J. (ed.) *Nephrology*, Chap. 36, pp. 583–594. (New York: John Wiley & Sons, Inc)
38. Hultengren, N. and Lagergren, C. (1965). A carcinoma of the renal pelvis in renal papillary necrosis. *Acta Chir. Scand.*, **130,** 314
39. Orell, S. R., Nanra, R. S. and Ferguson, N. W. (1979). Renal pelvic carcinoma in the Hunter Valley. *Med. J. Aust.*, **524,** 555–557
40. Bengtsson, U., Angervall, L., Ekman, H. and Lehmann, L. (1969). Transitional cell tumors of the renal pelvis in analgesic abusers. *Scand. J. Urol. Nephrol.*, **2,** 145–150
41. Taylor, J. S. (1972). Carcinoma of the urinary tract and analgesic abuse. *Med. J. Aust.*, **1,** 407
42. MacGregor, G. A., Jones, N. F., Barraclough, M. A., Wing, A. J. and Cranston, W. I. (1973). Ureteric stricture with analgesic nephropathy. *Br. Med. J.*, **2,** 271–272
43. McGregor, B., Saker, B. M. and England, E. J. (1979). Ureteric stricture associated with analgesic nephropathy. *Med. J. Aust.*, **1,** 287–288
44. Finan, B. F. and Finkbeiner, A. E. (1981). Renal papillary necrosis and retroperitoneal fibrosis secondary to analgesic abuse. *J. Urol*, **126,** 533–534

45. Weber, M., Braun, B. and Kohler, H. (1985). Ultrasonic findings in analgesic nephropathy. *Nephron*, **39,** 216–222
46. Lourie, S. H., Denman, S. J. and Schroder, E. T. (1977). Association of renal papillary necrosis and ankylosing spondylitis. *Arthritis Rheum.*, **20,** 917–921
47. Nanra, R. S., Hicks, J. D., McNamara, J. H., Lie, J. T., Leslie, D. W., Jackson, B. and Kincaid-Smith, P. (1970). Seasonal variation in the post-mortem incidence of renal papillary necrosis. *Med. J. Aust.*, **1,** 293–296
48. Wortmann, D. W., Kelsch, R. C., Kuhns, L., Sullivan, D. B. and Cassidy, J. T. (1980). Renal papillary necrosis in juvenile rheumatoid arthritis. *J. Pediatr.*, **97,** 37–40
49. Mitchell, H., Muirden, K. D. and Kincaid-Smith, P. (1982). Indomethacin-induced renal papillary necrosis in juvenile chronic arthritis. *Lancet*, **2,** 558–559
50. Morales, A. and Steyn, J. (1971). Papillary necrosis following phenylbutazone ingestion. *Arch. Surg.*, **103,** 420–421
51. Kincaid-Smith, P., Whitworth, J.A., Fairley, K. F. and Nanra, R. S. (1973). Clinical course of analgesic nephropathy with renal failure. In Haschek, H. (ed.) *Problems of Phenacetin Abuse*, p. 157. (Vienna: Facta Publications)
52. Berning, H., Orellana, K. and Selberg, W. (1974). Nieren papillen Nekrosen. *Deutsche Med. Wochenschrift*, **99,** 1749–1754
53. Prescott, L. F. (1982). Analgesic nephropathy: A reassessment of the role of phenacetin and other analgesics. *Drugs*, **23,** 75–149
54. Caruana, R. J. and Semble, E. (1984). Renal papillary necrosis due to naproxen. *J. Rheumatol.*, **11,** 90–91
55. Erwin, L. and Boulton Jones, J. M. (1982). Benoxaprofen and papillary necrosis. *Brit. Med. J.*, **285,** 694–695
56. Burry, H. C., Dieppe, P. A., Bresnihan, F. B. and Brown, C. (1976). Salicylates and renal function in rheumatoid arthritis. *Br. Med. J.*, **1,** 613–615
57. Murray, R. M., Lawson, D. H. and Linton, A. L. (1971). Analgesic nephropathy: clinical syndrome and prognosis. *Br. Med. J.*, **1,** 479–482
58. Bell, D., Kerr, D.N.S., Swinney, J. and Yeates, W. K. (1969). Analgesic nephropathy. Clinical course after withdrawal of phenacetin. *Brit. Med. J.*, **3,** 378–382
59. Gilman, A. (1964). Pharmacologic problems in evaluation of the role of analgesics in production of renal disease. In Kass, E. H. (ed.) *Progress in Pyelonephritis*, pp. 353–354. (Philadelphia: F. A. Davis Co.)
60. Nanra, R. S., Chirawong, P. and Kincaid-Smith, P. (1971). Renal papillary necrosis in rats produced by aspirin, APC and other analgesics. In Kincaid-Smith, P. and Fairley, K. F. (eds.) *Renal Infection and Renal Scarring*, pp. 385–400. (Melbourne: Mercedes Publishing Services)
61. Nanra, R. A. and Kincaid-Smith, P. (1973). Experimental renal papillary necrosis (RPN) with non-steroid anti-inflammatory analgesics. In Haschek H. (ed.) *Phenacetin Abuse 1973 – Internat. Symp. on Problems of Phenacetin Abuse, Vienna, 1973*, pp. 67–88. (Vienna: Facta Publications)
62. Wiseman, E. H. and Reinert, H. (1975). Anti-inflammatory drugs and renal papillary necrosis. *Agents Actions*, **5,** 322–325
63. Brown, D. M. and Hardy, T. L. (1968). Short-term study of the effect of phenacetin, phenazone and amidopyrine on the rat kidney. *Br. J. Pharmacol. Chemother.*, **32,** 17–24
64. Kaump, D. H. (1966). Pharmacology of the fenamates. II. Toxicology in animals. *Ann. Phys. Med.*, **9,** 16–23

65. Champion de Crespigny, P. J. and Kincaid-Smith, P. (1988). Caffeine aggravates mefenamic acid associated renal papillary damage. *Kidney Int.*, **33** (1), 135–136
66. Nanra, R. S. and Kincaid-Smith, P. (1970). Papillary necrosis in rats caused by aspirin and aspirin-containing mixtures. *Br. Med. J.*, **3,** 559–562
67. Wilson, D. R. and Gault, H. M. (1982). Declining incidence of analgesic nephropathy in Canada. *Can. Med. Assoc. J.*, **127,** 500–502
68. National Institutes of Health, Consensus Development Conference Statement (1984). *Analgesic-associated Kidney Disease.* US Department of Health and Human Services 5(2)
69. Segasothy, M. (1983). Analgesic use and abuse – a study in three selected population groups in Peninsular Malaysia. *Med. J. Malaysia*, **38,** 285–287
70. Segasothy, M., Kamal, A. and Suleiman, A. B. (1984). Renal papillary necrosis: retrospective radiological study. *Singapore Med. J.*, **25,** 254–258
71. Segasothy, M., Thyaparan, A., Siualingam, S., Kamal, A., Vijay, A. and Kumar, R. (1986). Renal papillary necrosis in Ipoh. *Med. J. Malaysia*, **41,** 19–23
72. Segasothy, M., Kamal, A., Das, D., Naidu, R. R. and Sivalingam, J. (1989). Renal papillary necrosis in the east coast of Peninsular Malaysia. *Med. J. Malaysia* (In press)
73. Segasothy, M., Kong, B. C. T., Kamal, A., Murad, Z. and Suleiman, A. B. (1983). Analgesic nephropathy – a prospective study. *Med. J. Malaysia*, **38,** 315–319
74. Segasothy, M., Cheong, I., King, B. C. T., Suleiman, A. B. and Morad, Z. (1986). Further evidence of analgesic nephropathy in Malaysia. *Med. J. Malaysia*, **41,** 377–379
75. Segasothy, M., Suleiman, A. B., Puvaneswary, M. and Rohana, A. (1989). Paracetamol: A cause for analgesic nephropathy and end-stage renal disease. *Nepron* (in press)
76. Michielson, P., van Damme, B., Dotremont, G., Verberckmoes, R., Oei, L. S. and Vermylen, J. (1973). Indomethacin treatment of membranoproliferative and lobular glomerulonephritis. In Kincaid-Smith, P., Mathews, D. and Becker, G. (eds.) *Glomerulonephritis*, pp. 611–631. (New York: John Wiley & Sons)
77. Kimberly, R. P. and Plotz, P. H. (1977). Aspirin-induced depression of renal function. *N. Engl. J. Med.*, **296,** 418–424
78. Arisz, L., Donker, A. J. M., Brentjens, J. R. H. and van der Hem, G. K. (1976). The effect of indomethacin on proteinuria and kidney function in the nephrotic syndrome. *Acta Med. Scand.*, **199,** 121–125
79. Kleinknecht, C., Broyer, M., Gubler, M. C. and Palcoux, J. B. (1980). Irreversible renal failure after indomethacin in steroid-resistant nephrosis. *N. Engl. J. Med.*, **302,** 691
80. Tan, S. Y., Shapiro, R. and Kish, M. A. (1979). Reversible acute renal failure induced by indomethacin. *J. Am. Med. Assoc.*, **241,** 2732–2733
81. Fawaz-Estrup, F. and Ho, G. Jr. (1981). Reversible acute renal failure induced by indomethacin. *Arch. Int. Med.*, **141,** 1670–1671
82. Findling, J. W., Beckstrom, D., Rawsthorne, L., Kozin, F. and Itskovitz, H. (1980). Indomethacin-induced hyperkalemia in three patients with gouty arthritis. *J. Am. Med. Assoc.*, **244,** 1127–1128
83. Galler, M., Folkert, V. W. and Scholondorff, D. (1981). Reversible acute renal insufficiency and hyperkalemia following indomethacin therapy. *J. Am. Med. Assoc.*, **246,** 154–155

84. Cibattoni, G., Pugliese, F., Cinotti, G. A. and Patrono, C. (1980). Renal effects of anti-inflammatory drugs. *Eur. J. Rheum. Inflamm.*, **3,** 210–221
85. Ciabattoni, G., Cinotti, G. A., Pierucci, A., Simonetti, B. M., Manzi, M., Pugliese, F., Barsotti, P., Pecci, G., Jaggi, F. and Patrono, C. (1984). Effects of sulindac and ibuprofen in patients with chronic glomerular disease: Evidence for the dependence of renal function on prostacyclin. *N. Engl. J. Med.*, **310,** 279–283
86. Kimberly, R. P., Sherman, R. L., Mouradian, J. and Lockshin, M. D. (1979). Apparent acute renal failure associated with therapeutic aspirin and ibuprofen administration. *Arthritis Rheum.*, **22,** 281–285
87. Donker, A. J. M., Arisz, L., Brentjens, J. R. H., van der Hem, G. K. and Hollemans, H. J. G. (1976). The effect of indomethacin on kidney function and plasma renin activity in man. *Nephron*, **17,** 288–296
88. Walsh, J. J. and Venuto, R. C. (1979). Acute oliguric renal failure induced by indomethacin: Possible mechanisms. *Ann. Int. Med.*, **91,** 47–49
89. Boyer, T. D., Zia, P. and Reynold, T. B. (1979). Effect of indomethacin and prostaglandin A1 on renal function and plasma renin activity in alcoholic liver disease. *Gastroenterology*, **77,** 215
90. Zipser, R. D., Hoefs, J. C., Speckart, P. F., Dia, P. K. and Horton, R. (1979). Prostaglandins: Modulators of renal function and pressor resistance in chronic liver disease. *J. Clin. Endocrinol. Metab.*, **49,** 895–900
91. Fairley, K. F., Woo, K. T., Birch, D. F., Leaker, B. R. and Ratnaike, S. (1986). Triamterene induced crystalluria and cylinduria: clinical and experimental studies (Dytac or Dyazide). *Clin. Nephrol.*, **26**(4), 169–173
92. Goldszer, R. C., Coodley, E. L., Rosner, M. J., Simons, W. M. and Schwartz, A. B. (1981). Hyperkalaemia associated with indomethacin. *Arch. Int. Med.*, **141,** 802–804
93. Berionade, V., Corneille, L. and Haraoui, B. (1979). Indomethacin-induced inhibition of prostaglandin with hyperkalemia. *Ann. Int. Med.*, **19,** 499–500
94. Kutyrina, I. M., Androsova, S. O. and Tareyeva, I. E. (1979). Indomethacin-induced hyporeninaemic hypoaldosteronism. *Lancet*, **1,** 785
95. Paladini, G. and Tonazzi, C. (1982). Indomethacin-induced hyperkalemia and renal failure in multiple myeloma. *Acta Haematol.*, **68,** 256–260
96. Tan, S. Y., Shapiro, R., Franco, R., Stockard, H. and Mulro, P. J. (1979). Indomethacin-induced prostaglandin inhibition with hyperkalemia: A reversible cause of hyporeninemic hypoaldosteronism. *Ann. Int. Med.*, **90,** 783–785
97. Halliday, H. L., Hirata, T. and Brady, J. P. (1979). Indomethacin therapy for large patent ductus arteriosus in the very low birth weight infant: Results and complications. *Pediatrics*, **64,** 154–159
98. Blackshear, J. L., Davidman, M. and Stillman, T. (1983). Identification of risk from renal insufficiency from non-steroidal anti-inflammatory drugs. *Arch. Int. Med.*, **143,** 1130–1134
99. Garella, S. and Matanese, R. A. (1984). Renal effects of prostaglandins and clinical adverse effects of non-steroidal anti-inflammatory agents. *Medicine (Baltimore)*, **63,** 165–181
100. Fong, H. J. and Cohen, A. H. (1982). Ibuprofen-induced acute renal failure with acute tubular necrosis. *Am. J. Nephrol.*, **2,** 28–31
101. Lipsett, M. B. and Goldman, R. (1954). Phenylbutazone toxicity: Report of a case of acute renal failure. *Ann. Intern. Med.*, **41,** 1075–1079

102. McDonald, F. D., Lazarus, G. S. and Campbell, W. L. (1982). Phenylbutazone anuria. *South. Med. J.*, **60,** 1318–1320
103. Weisman, J. I. and Bloom, B. (1955). Anuria following phenylbutazone therapy. *N. Engl. J. Med.*, **252,** 1086–1087
104. Boelaert, J., van Eeghem, P., Daneels, R., Schurgers, M., Fagard, R., Lijnen, P., Verschueren, L. J. and Amery, A. (1981). Renal dysfunction due to anturane. *N. Engl. J. Med.*, **305,** 1154
105. Braun, J. (1976). Abnormalities of urinary sediment and renal failure following sulfinpyrazone therapy. *Arch. Intern. Med.*, **136,** 1060–1061
106. Butler, A. L. (1981). Renal dysfunction due to anturane. *N. Engl. J. Med.*, **305,** 106
107. Docci, D., Durci, F. and Salvi, G. (1983). Sulfinpyrazone-associated acute renal failure. *Clin. Nephrol.*, **20,** 53–54
108. Howard, T., Hoy, R. H., Warren, S., Georgieu, M. and Selinger, H. (1981). Acute renal dysfunction due to sulfinpyrazone therapy in post-myocardial infarction cardiomegaly: Reversible hypersensitive interstitial nephritis. *Am. Heart J.*, **102,** 294–295
109. Bennett, W. M., Van Zee, B. E. and Hutchings, R. (1979). Acute renal failure from ticrynafen. *N. Engl. J. Med*, **301,** 1179
110. Cohen, L. H., Norby, L. H., Champion, C. and Spargo, B. (1979). Acute renal failure with ticrynafen. *N. Engl. J. Med.*, **301,** 1180
111. Walker, R. G., Whitworth, J. A. and Kincaid-Smith, P. (1980). Acute interstitial nephritis in a patient taking tielinic acid. *Br. Med. J.*, **280,** (6225), 1212
112. Robertson, C.E., Ford, M. J. H., Van Someren, V., Dlugolecka, M. and Prescott, J. F. (1980). Mefenamic acid nephropathy. *Lancet*, **2,** 232–233
113. Venning, V., Dixon, A. J. and Oliver, D. O. (1980). Mefenamic acid nephropathy. *Lancet*, **2,** 745–746
114. Malik, S., Arthurton, I. and Griffiths, I. D. (1980). Mefenamic acid nephropathy. *Lancet*, **2,** 746
115. Brandstetter, R. D. and Mar, D. D. (1978). Reversible oliguric renal failure associated with ibuprofen treatment. *Br. Med. J.*, **2,** 1194–1195
116. Bernheim, J. L. and Korzets, Z. (1979). Indomethacin-induced renal failure. *Ann. Intern. Med.*, **91,** 792
117. Bunning, R. D. and Barth, W. F. (1982). Sulindac. A potentially renal-sparing nonsteroidal anti-inflammatory drug. *J. Am. Med. Assoc.*, **248,** 2864–2867
118. Favre, L., Glasson, P. and Vallotton, M. B. (1982). Reversible acute renal failure from combined triamterene and indomethacin: A study in healthy subjects. *Ann. Intern. Med.*, **96,** 317–320
119. Lomvardias, S., Pinn, V. W., Wadhawa, M. L., Koshy, K. M. and Heller, M. (1981). Nephrotic syndrome associated with sulindac. *N. Engl. J. Med.*, **304,** 424
120. Cartwright, K. C., Trotter, T. L. and Cohen, M. L. (1979). Naproxen nephrotoxicity. *Arizona Med.*, **36,** 124–126
121. Katz, S. M., Capaldo, R., Everts, E. A. and Di Gregorio, J. G. (1981). Tolmetin: Association with reversible renal failure and acute interstitial nephritis. *J. Am. Med. Assoc.*, **246,** 243–245
122. McCarthy, J. T., Schwarts, G. L., Blair, T. J., Pierides, A. M. and Van Der Berg, C. J. (1982). Reversible nonoliguric acute renal failure associated with zomepirac therapy. *Mayo Clin. Proc.*, **57,** 351–354

123. Russell, G. I., Bing, R. F., Walls, J. and Pettigre, N. M. (1978). Interstitial nephritis in a case of phenylbutazone hypersensitivity. *Br. Med. J.*, **1,** 1322
124. Woods, K. L. and Michael, J. (1981). Mefenamic acid nephropathy. *Brit. Med. J.*, **282,** 1471
125. Bender, W. L., Bexhorner, W. E., Hall-Craggs, H., Whelton, A. and Solez, K. (1983). Specificity of the renal lesion of fenoprofen nephropathy. *Clin. Res.*, **31,** 424A
126. Brezin, J. P., Katz, S. M., Schwartz, A. B. and Chinitz, J. L. (1979). Reversible renal failure and nephrotic syndrome associated with nonsteroidal anti-inflammatory agents. *N. Engl. J. Med.*, **301,** 1271–1273
127. Chatterjee, G. P. (1981). Nephrotic syndrome induced by tolmetin. *J. Am. Med. Assoc.*, **246,** 1589
128. Curt, G. A., Kaldany, A., Whitley, L. G., Crosson, A. W., Rolla, A., Merino, M. J. and d'Elia, J. (1980). Reversible rapidly progressive renal failure with nephrotic syndrome due to fenoprofen calcium. *Ann. Intern. Med.*, **92,** 72–73
129. Finkelstein, A., Fraley, D. S., Stachura, I., Feldman, H. A., Gandy, D. R. and Bourke, E. (1982). Fenoprofen nephropathy: Lipoid nephrosis and interstitial nephritis. A possible T-lymphocyte disorder. *Am. J. Med.*, **72,** 81–87
130. Gary, N. E., Dodelson, R. and Eisinger, R. P. (1980). Indomethacin-associated acute renal failure. *Am. J. Med.*, **69,** 135–136
131. Handa, S. P. (1980). Renal effects of fenoprofen. *Ann. Intern. Med.*, **93,** 508
132. Joshi, S. J. and Stern, K. (1982). Spontaneous recovery of nephrotic syndrome associated with tolmetin. (Abstract) *Am. Soc. Nephrol.*, **12,** 34A
133. Lorch, J., Lefavour, G., Davidson, H. and Cortell, S. (1980). Renal effects of fenoprofen. *Ann. Intern. Med.*, **93,** 509
134. Miller, R. T., Anderson, R. J., Linas, S. L. *et al.* (1978). Urinary diagnostic indices in acute renal failure. A prospective study. *Ann. Intern. Med.*, **89,** 47
135. Piper, P. J. and Vane, R. J. (1969). Release of additional factors in anaphylaxis and its antagonism by anti-inflammatory drugs. *Nature (London)*, **223,** 29
136. Stachura, I., Jayakumar, S. and Bourke, E. (1983). T and B lymphocyte subsets in fenoprofen nephropathy. *Am. J. Med.*, **75,** 9–16
137. Wendland, M. L., Wagoner, R. A. and Holley, K. E. (1980). Renal failure associated with fenoprofen. *Mayo Clin. Proc.*, **55,** 103–107
138. Clive, D. M. and Stoff, J. D. S. (1984). Renal syndromes associated with nonsteroidal anti-inflammatory drugs. *N. Engl. J. Med.*, **301,** 563–571
139. Kincaid-Smith, P. (1986). Effects of non-narcotic analgesics on the kidney. *Drugs*, **32** (4), 109–128
140. Prescott, L. F. (1982). Analgesic nephropathy: A reassessment of the role of phenacetin and other analgesics. *Drugs*, **23,** 75–149
141 Nanra, R. S. and Kincaid-Smith, P. (1975). Renal papillary necrosis in rheumatoid arthritis. *Med. J. Aust.*, **1,** 194–197
142 Nanra, R. S. and Kincaid-Smith, P. (1973). Experimental and clinical analgesic nephropathy with aspirin. In Haschek, H. (ed.) *Problems of Phenacetin Abuse*, pp. 89–114. (Vienna: Facta Publications)

2

INTERSTITIAL NEPHRITIS

C. G. NEWSTEAD and F. P. MARSH

In this chapter, we shall discuss the histological features, clinical presentation, putative mechanisms, clinical management and prognosis of drug-induced tubulo-interstitial nephritis (TIN). Analgesic-induced TIN (discussed in Chapter 1) and TIN which is not due to drugs are outside the scope of this article.

HISTOLOGICAL FEATURES

In interstitial nephritis the cardinal pathological abnormality consists of inflammatory cell infiltration of the interstitium, although tubular damage is also evident. A pronounced cellular reaction is often found in typical acute tubular necrosis but it is usually possible to differentiate histologically between these two diagnoses. In acute TIN, the glomeruli are normal, becoming sclerosed only in chronic cases.

Because of the histological overlap between cases presenting acutely and those of an apparently chronic nature, the distinction between acute and chronic interstitial nephritis tends to be made clinically rather than histologically, and, in particular, relates to the speed of onset of renal failure. In patients where this is rapid, the interstitial infiltrate generally consists of acute inflammatory cells, often eosinophilic, but sometimes plasma cells predominate and oedema may be marked. In patients with a chronic presentation the cellular infiltrate tends to be lymphocytic, interstitial oedema is not marked and fibrosis may be prominent. However, the histological overlap is considerable and lymphocytes and plasma cells may predominate in acute cases. The development of interstitial fibrosis is an important indicator of chronicity.

The histology gives little indication of the cause of the nephropathy and similar appearances may be found, for example, in acute TIN attributed to drugs, infection, acute transplant rejection, generalized conditions, such as systemic lupus erythematosus, and in idiopathic TIN. Likewise, the histological changes of chronic TIN, which may evolve following acute TIN with continued drug exposure[1], give little indication of the original cause. Similar changes may be found in chronic TIN associated with obstructive uropathy, pyelonephritis, ischaemia, sarcoidosis, Sjögren's syndrome, Balkan nephropathy, radiation injury, medullary cystic disease and chronic renal transplant rejection.

INCIDENCE OF ACUTE DRUG-INDUCED TIN

Although drugs are increasingly considered as an important cause of acute renal failure (ARF)[2,3], the incidence of drug-induced TIN is uncertain because of incomplete notification, insecure diagnoses and because the population exposed to individual drugs is difficult to quantify. Even the proportion of patients with ARF who have drug-induced TIN is difficult to determine. Comprehensive data come from Richet *et al.*[4] who performed renal biopsies in 218 of 976 patients presenting with ARF: only 8 (3.6%) of those biopsied (0.8% of the whole group) were thought to have drug-induced TIN. Patients not subjected to biopsy were considered likely on clinical grounds to have acute tubular necrosis rather than TIN but as this was not established histologically the true frequency of TIN probably exceeded 0.8%. In contrast, in a more recent large multicentre study of 2175 patients with ARF, drugs were implicated as the cause in 398 (18.3%); TIN was found in 17 of 77 renal biopsies (22%) but the criteria for biopsy and for the diagnosis of a drug-induced causation were not specified clearly[5]. In 84 unselected patients with ARF who underwent renal biopsy, 10% had acute TIN[6]. Sixteen percent of 80 children treated with methicillin developed an acute allergic reaction with reversible renal failure in an unbiopsied series collected over ten years[7]. Likewise,

Nolan and Abernathy[8] found haematuria and proteinuria, usually with eosinophilia, in nine of 52 patients (17%) treated with methicillin for staphylococcal bacteraemia; five developed reversible renal failure. The high frequency may relate to the prolonged therapy given, although it is possible that the combination of staphylococcal bacteraemia and methicillin treatment is associated with a particularly high incidence of TIN. Only one of 29 similar patients treated with cephalosporins was affected in the same way. In a review of over 150 cases of methicillin-associated TIN[9] 33% had received the drug for over three weeks and 75% for more than a month, although typical cases can occur after much shorter courses of treatment. Many reports of drug-induced nephrotoxicity refer to methicillin and other β-lactam antibiotics[2,9–28]. Other common causes of acute TIN include rifampicin, co-trimoxazole, thiazides, frusemide and phenindione. Sulphonamides have long been implicated[29,30]. Thiazides and frusemide are structurally related to sulphonamides and are increasingly reported to cause biopsy-proven TIN[31,32]. Over 60 cases have been attributed to rifampicin[33,34] and 30 to phenindione[35]. See Table 2.1 for the frequency of TIN associated with individual drugs.

In summary, the true incidence of drug-induced TIN is not possible to determine because of selective and retrospective data recording, uncontrolled series and diagnoses made on the basis of clinical suspicion without biopsy confirmation. Patients with ARF tend to be labelled as having drug-induced TIN when an agent known to cause this condition has been prescribed recently, although the connection may be fortuitous.

CLINICAL PRESENTATION

Acute drug-induced TIN

The clinical features of acute drug-induced TIN classically begin abruptly with fever (85–100% of patients) and macroscopic or microscopic haematuria (95%)[18]. About one third of patients report overt haematuria. A maculopapular rash, often itchy, is seen in 25–50% of patients. Sterile pyuria, mild proteinuria (less than 2 g/24 h) and eosinophiluria are often found[26]. Eosinophilia, typically lasting only one to two days, occurs in 80%[27]. There may be evidence of tubular

TABLE 2.1 Frequency of TIN associated with individual drugs

Frequent	
***	Co-trimoxazole
***	Frusemide
***	Methicillin
***	Phenindione
***	Rifampicin
***	Sulphonamides
***	Thiazides
Rare	
***	Allopurinol
***	Amoxycillin
***	Ampicillin
***	Carbenicillin
**	Cefoxitin
***	Cephalexin
***	Cephalothin
***	Cephradine
***	Cimetidine
***	Lithium
***	Nafcillin
***	Oxacillin
***	Penicillin G
***	Phenytoin
***	Sulphinpyrazone
***	Cisplatin
Isolated case reports	
**	Captopril[127]
***	Carbamazepine[128]
***	Clofibrate[129]
**	Gentamicin[57]
***	Interferon[130]
***	Minocycline[131]
***	Radiological contrast agents[132]
***	Tienilic acid[133]
*	Vancomycin[134]
***	Erythromycin[135]

*** Clinical evidence of systemic allergic phenomenon plus biopsy-proven TIN
** Similar clinical evidence, *no* biopsy
* Dubious clinical evidence, no biopsy
See body of text for main references

impairment[10,27], with glycosuria, aminoaciduria, sodium wasting, renal tubular acidosis and (rarely) potassium conservation[36]. The classical triad of rash, fever and eosinophilia is seen in less than 30% of patients[37] and acute drug-induced TIN can occur in the absence of any of these clinical features. It should, therefore, be suspected in any case of ARF of unknown aetiology and early renal biopsy is helpful in confirming the presence of interstitial nephritis.

Chronic drug-induced TIN

There are no particular symptoms which distinguish chronic drug-induced TIN from other causes of chronic renal failure. Because of this, and because the diagnosis of chronic TIN is uncertain in the absence of renal biopsy, its relationship to current and previously prescribed drugs may be impossible to determine in individual patients. The contribution of chronic TIN to end-stage renal failure is uncertain.

REVIEW OF REPORTS OF DRUG-ASSOCIATED TIN

Sulphonamides

Although sulphonamides have been used clinically for over 50 years, proven TIN has been attributed to them only infrequently. They were, however, among the first drugs to be clearly associated with the condition[29,30]. These initial reports were based upon postmortem histology. In the first report of 78 deaths after sulphonamide treatment for various serious medical conditions, interstitial nephritis was present in about 50% of cases. More *et al.* reviewed 2000 postmortem examinations. In 375 cases, there was known exposure to sulphonamides antemortem; interstitial nephritis was seen in 11 cases[30]. Robson *et al.*[38] described two cases. In the first, renal biopsy appearances of tubulo-interstitial nephritis were associated with a high circulating IgE concentration. In the second, a 10-day course of sulphadiazine, given for urinary tract infection, led to oliguria requiring dialysis for six weeks. Biopsy revealed acute tubulo-interstitial nephritis; 17 days later a repeat biopsy showed more extensive changes and increased interstitial oedema. Treatment with prednisolone (40 mg daily) appeared to cause an almost immediate increase in urinary volume. Although, three months later, creatinine clearance was 65 ml/min, a further renal biopsy showed marked interstitial fibrosis.

The frequency of sulphonamide-induced TIN has increased recently due to the frequent prescription of co-trimoxazole[2,3,40–47]. In 16 patients, 14 of whom had previously normal renal function, acute non-oliguric reversible renal failure was precipitated by co-trimoxazole given in normal or reduced dose[41]. In two patients, who did not have pre-existing renal disease, biopsy showed 'acute tubular necrosis' with interstitial oedema and cellular infiltration. Co-trimoxazole was implicated because of the prompt recovery of function which followed withdrawal of the drug. An apparent response to prednisolone in three cases, and recurrence of the condition in one who was again given co-trimoxazole (leading to irreversible loss of renal function), suggests that TIN rather than acute tubular necrosis, was the likely diagnosis in them also.

Methicillin

Acute interstitial nephritis due to methicillin has been described on many occasions[2,9–18,20–29,36]. In one early report[10], four patients treated with methicillin and four others given benzylpenicillin in high dose for a prolonged period developed uraemia and eosinophilia; a rash occurred in four and pyrexia in six. Interstitial nephritis was noted histologically in the four patients subjected to renal biopsy. Renal function and urinary sediment returned to normal between three and 32 days after stopping the antibiotic, although one patient died. Recovery, when it occurs, may not be rapid. In one case[12], acute renal failure, eosinophilia and haematuria developed during methicillin treatment and the patient required regular haemodialysis for two months after the antibiotic was withdrawn and prednisolone therapy started. Renal biopsy obtained a fortnight after withdrawal of the antibiotic showed classical TIN. IgG, C3 and 'methicillin antigen' were deposited linearly on the tubular basement membrane (but not on the glomerular basement membrane), the hypothesis being that a tubular basement membrane protein formed a hapten–protein conjugate with methicillin, stimulating antibody formation.

Methicillin-induced TIN is said to be much more common in males than in females (relative incidence 3:1)[13] but, in children, the sex and age distribution is uncertain. Review of the literature does not suggest that the development of the condition is dose dependent, except for those reports of methicillin-induced TIN in patients with staphylococcal septicaemia; it has been described as early as two days and as late as 37 days after the start of treatment. Fever has been described in 87% of cases, eosinophilia in 79%, haematuria (gross or microscopic) in 97%, proteinuria in 94% and pyuria in 93%, usually with eosinophiluria[13]. Overt haematuria[18] is relatively common. In another series, eosinophilia occurred in all 14 patients described, and eosinophiluria was also frequently present[26], a rash occurring in about a quarter of cases.

Renal failure of sufficient severity to require dialysis support appears to be relatively common in adults (30%) but is rare in children under 16 years old[13].

Rifampicin

Acute renal failure associated with the intermittent use of rifampicin has often been described[24,42–51]. It has also occurred in patients allegedly taking daily rifampicin[52] although their compliance with treatment must remain uncertain. The danger of resuming rifampicin after an interval is well recognized and, after a period without the drug, even a single dose can cause reversible oliguric renal failure requiring dialysis[42]. In this case, renal biopsy showed normal glomeruli and tubules with interstitial oedema and lymphocytic infiltration. In two patients given a single dose after treatment had been stopped for four or five days, fever, myalgia, nausea, diarrhoea and oliguria developed within a few hours. Anuria lasted three days in one patient, nine days in the other and recovery was incomplete in one of the cases[43]. A similar acute illness occurred in a patient who accidentally took one dose of rifampicin after treatment had been stopped for two months[43]. Within 30 minutes, he experienced lumbar pain, fever, chills and arthralgia followed by vomiting, diarrhoea and anuria. There was no eosinophilia, but renal biopsy showed patchy necrosis and flattened proximal tubular epithelium, marked interstitial oedema, mononuclear infiltration and fibrosis. The glomeruli were normal on light and immunofluorescent microscopy.

Rarely, symptoms develop in patients taking regular twice weekly rifampicin: malaise, fever, rigors and reversible renal failure were reported in only one of 49 patients so treated[45]. A treatment gap of as little as four days has led to vomiting, diarrhoea, lumbar pain, chills and oliguria with eosinophilia and biopsy evidence of interstitial nephritis. In this case, immunofluorescent microscopy was normal[46]. Oliguria persisted for nine days despite treatment with prednisolone but there was full recovery of renal function.

Renal biopsies[30,42–44,46] have demonstrated interstitial oedema, inflammatory cell infiltrates and tubular necrosis but the glomeruli remain normal. Because rifampicin can induce antibodies[45], and because rifampicin–antibody complexes can bind to erythrocytes and induce a haemolytic anaemia, it has been suggested that the renal failure may be caused by immune complexes[44]. This theory, however, remains unproven. Antibodies to rifampicin can be detected with the same frequency in patients who do not develop ARF as in those who do.

Phenindione

Acute TIN used to develop relatively frequently in patients treated with this oral anticoagulant[53,54], but it is now rarely prescribed. The clinical presentation was similar to that of methicillin nephritis but hepatitis often occurred also. The mortality was high and interstitial fibrosis developed in some of the survivors[55].

Diuretics

Thiazides and frusemide are structurally related to sulphonamides and it is, therefore, not surprising that they also can cause acute TIN. Chlorthalidone[55], hydrochlorothiazide[2,56], bendrofluazide[57], triamterene[58] and frusemide[31,59–61] have all been incriminated, as have combined preparations: chlorthalidone–hydrochlorothiazide[59], hydrochlorthalidone–triamterene[3,32,60,61] and triamterene–frusemide[47].

Penicillins

Apart from methicillin (see p. 42), these have not often been reported as causing TIN. Benzyl penicillin has rarely been incriminated[10,62]. Colvin[62] reported a patient with bacterial endocarditis who developed low grade fever, eosinophilia, eosinophiluria and progressive non-oliguric renal failure during the fourth week of treatment with benzyl penicillin. Renal biopsy demonstrated an intense interstitial infiltrate. Using indirect immunofluorescence, rabbit antiserum to benzyl penicillin bound to the interstitium and to tubular basement membranes. This observation, however, is not necessarily of pathogenic significance, because it has been found in patients without renal disease who died whilst taking penicillin.

Ampicillin has been associated with TIN more often than benzyl penicillin[15,20,63–65], and interstitial oedema and inflammatory infiltrates with normal glomerular morphology have been recorded[63,64]. Amoxycillin[66], oxycillin[28,67,68] and nafcillin[28,69] have also been incriminated. The presentation is usually less acute in its development than that classically induced by rifampicin but this is not invariable. In one 12-year-old patient[64] the clinical course was reminiscent of that due to rifampicin: one hour after the first dose of ampicillin prescribed for skin sepsis, the patient became ill with fever, nausea, vomiting, eosinophilia and proteinuria. Although renal function remained normal, renal biopsy was consistent with interstitial nephritis. The patient had been exposed to penicillin some six years previously without adverse reaction.

Typical clinical and histological features of TIN have occurred following prolonged carbenicillin therapy[70,71]; immunochemical staining was unremarkable.

Cephalosporins

As these drugs are structurally related to penicillin, it is not surprising that cephalothin[72–74] and cephradine[75] have also been reported to cause TIN. Cross-sensitization with penicillin derivatives has been described[3,76] although there was no recurrence in one patient with cephalosporin-induced TIN who was subsequently challenged with penicillin[77].

Intravenous cefoxitin, given after limb amputation for gangrene, was reported to cause acute renal failure, eosinophilia and haematuria: spontaneous recovery occurred following withdrawal of the drug but dialysis was necessary; there was no biopsy[78]. Cephalexin was thought to be the cause in one patient who developed renal failure after methicillin and gentamicin treatment of staphylococcal sepsis was changed to cephalexin. A renal biopsy revealed acute tubulo-interstitial nephritis as well as glomerulonephritis. The patient recovered after withdrawal of cephalexin and the prescription of steroid therapy[73].

Lithium

Hestbech *et al.*[79] compared renal biopsies from 14 normotensive patients undergoing prolonged lithium treatment with histology from age-matched controls. In the patients, who all had nephrogenic diabetes insipidus or a history of acute lithium intoxication, interstitial infiltration, fibrosis and tubular atrophy were significantly more common. Immunofluorescent studies were negative. The only prolonged psychotropic medication taken by the patients had been lithium and no other causative factors could be identified.

The same group[80] questioned the safety of long-term lithium treatment in a study (from the one psychiatric clinic) of 110 patients treated with lithium for more than 6 months. Thirty-two had abnormal renal function. Renal biopsy in 14 of 18 subjects considered likely, on clinical grounds, to have lithium-induced nephropathy, showed findings similar to those in their earlier study. At least 25% of the patients who had taken lithium for more than 2 years had developed a chronic nephropathy characterized by impaired renal concentrating ability; in a few, modest increases in serum creatinine had occurred.

Functional changes suggestive of chronic lithium-induced nephropathy were also found by Bucht and Wahlin[81]. In patients undergoing long-term therapy, impaired concentrating capacity was also noted in those taking neuroleptics alone, although it was most marked if both neuroleptics and lithium were taken. The appropriateness in

Hestbech's *et al* (1977) study[79] of using controls who were not taking any psychotropics is, therefore, questionable. Chronic interstitial fibrosis has been described in psychiatric patients not taking lithium[82].

Phenytoin

Isolated TIN has been less frequently reported than a systemic allergic response with renal vasculitis[52,83–85]. In one patient, who developed fever, rash and eosinophilia 22 days after the onset of phenytoin therapy, renal biopsy confirmed TIN. There was linear immunofluorescence along the renal tubular basement membrane on which deposits of diphenylhydantoin could be demonstrated.

Allopurinol

This drug has been described as causing TIN as well as glomerulonephritis, vasculitis, hepatitis, skin rashes and generalized allergic disorders[86–89]. However, the attribution is not secure. In one report[87], the course was suggestive of systemic allergic vasculitis rather than TIN and the patient, who had been treated with several drugs, was not biopsied. Fever, oliguria, eosinophilia and histologically proven TIN were attributed to allopurinol in another case[88] who was also receiving colchicine. In a further publication[86], oliguric acute renal failure was attributed to allopurinol as part of a multisystem disorder, but in one of the two patients biopsied the effects were more consistent with a vasculitis.

Cimetidine

The first case report concerned a 22-year-old male who, after two weeks' treatment with cimetidine, developed fever, myalgia, sterile pyuria, proteinuria and renal impairment. Biopsy showed changes of interstitial nephritis. Five months after withdrawal of the drug, his renal function had returned to normal[90]. In a second case, sterile pyuria and renal failure developed during exposure to the drug for a second time. The symptoms improved following withdrawal of treatment, but inadvertent retreatment with cimetidine on a third occasion led to recurrence of the fever, proteinuria and pyuria after one day[91]. Another case occurred in a man treated with cimetidine for 11 months. He presented with severe non-oliguric renal failure, myalgia, proximal muscle weakness, sterile pyuria and eosinophilia. Urinary protein excretion was 1.3 g/24 h and serum phosphocreatine kinase was elevated. Biopsies showed changes of interstitial nephritis and a polymyositis. Haemodialysis support was required. One week after withdrawal of cimetidine and a trial of prednisolone, serum creatinine had fallen to near normal[92].

Richman *et al.*[93] reported a patient who developed fever and biopsy-proven acute interstitial nephritis and tubulitis a week after the introduction of cimetidine. Immunofluorescent studies on the kidneys were negative; haemodialysis was required. Serum creatinine fell to 240 mmol/l with 80 mg prednisolone daily but deteriorated when the steroid was tapered. Marked improvement occurred after the withdrawal of cimetidine and with a temporary increase in steroid dosage.

Platinum

Focal necrosis and tubular dilatation has been described following cisplatin treatment[94–96]. The severity of renal impairment is closely related to the total dose and the histological changes can progress to chronic TIN[94].

PATHOGENESIS OF TIN

The pathogenesis of drug-induced TIN in humans is unknown. Animal models of immunological disturbances which can produce TIN fall into three categories[97]

(1) Immune complex deposition in the interstitium or on tubular basement membranes.
(2) Antitubular basement membrane antibody formation.
(3) Cell-mediated immune mechanisms.

Immune complex deposition

In the same way that animal models of immune complex glomerulonephritis have been studied following the injection of kidney extracts, an immune complex TIN characterized by immunoglobulin and complement deposition along the TBM can be induced in rabbits by the injection of rabbit kidney extracts in conjunction with adjuvant[98,99]. Exogenous antigens (bovine[100] or human[101] albumin) injected repeatedly into rabbits can result in chronic serum sickness nephritis with granular deposits along the TBM as well as in the glomeruli. Apart from the mononuclear cell infiltrate produced, these models appear to have little in common with, and shed little light on, the human pathophysiology.

Changes more comparable with those found in human drug-induced TIN may be produced in rats by the repeated injection of Tamm-Horsfall protein (THP)[102–104]. In this model, deposits of THP, IgG and C3 are found along the TBM of the cells of the ascending limb but not in the glomeruli, together with an interstitial inflammatory reaction.

Although an immune complex interstitial nephritis may be found in SLE[105,106] and occasionally immune aggregates have been found along the TBM in cases of 'idiopathic' human TIN[107,108], the relevance of this pathogenetic mechanism to human drug-induced TIN is not clear.

Anti-TBM antibody formation

Although, in humans, anti-TBM antibodies may play a role in Goodpasture's syndrome, some glomerulonephropathies and in transplant glomerulopathy, the number of cases in which they have been implicated in TIN is very small. In some cases of methicillin nephritis[10,12], a linear fluorescence was seen along the TBM and the serum contained antibodies directed against dimethoxyphenylpenicillinoyl hapten bound to the TBM. Anti-TBM antibodies in other drug-induced TIN have rarely been isolated[29,97,98,103].

Experimentally, tubular damage and mononuclear and giant cell infiltration of the interstitium develop in guinea pigs injected with rabbit TBM and Freund's adjuvant. Guinea pig IgG is deposited linearly along the TBM, and anti-TBM antibodies are present in the blood[109]. In guinea pigs injected with bovine renal basement membrane fraction, linear deposition of IgG can be found on TBM, and often also on glomerular basement membrane. Antibodies eluted from the kidneys possess both anti-TBM and anti-GBM activity[110].

Rats develop a mononuclear interstitial reaction, with linear deposition of IgG and C3 along the TBM, after injection with rat kidney, Freund's adjuvant and pertussis vaccine[111] or bovine TBM and pertussis[112]. Anti-TBM antibodies from the serum of an injected animal can produce an interstitial nephritis in a second animal, with the development of interstitial fibrosis and chronic tubular damage. Passive transfer of the disease in guinea pigs is impossible if the recipients are depleted of complement with cobra venom[113], although anti-TBM antibody can be produced in guinea pigs lacking C4[114]. The initial event in these models is presumed to be the binding of anti-TBM antibody to the TBM with cell-mediated immunity implicated as a necessary secondary phase. Further evidence for the amplifying role of cell-mediated immunity comes from guinea pig models of TIN initiated by anti-TBM antibodies and in which mononuclear cells are dominant in the interstitium. Their bone marrow origin was shown when injections of anti-TBM antibody into animals whose bone marrows had been destroyed by radiation did not lead to TIN. However, injection of bone marrow cells from normal guinea pigs into the animals that had been irradiated and had also received injections of foreign TBM allowed TIN to develop[115].

Cell-mediated mechanisms

Although there is no firm evidence that cell-mediated mechanisms are important in the production of human TIN, they have been implicated in animal models. In guinea pigs[116] and rats[117], TIN has been produced and transferred to naive animals by spleen or lymph node cells, but not by serum; there was no evidence of anti-TBM antibodies nor of immune deposits on the tubules. In a spontaneous murine model of TIN, cell transfer proved possible using cells with a cytotoxic T cell phenotype[118]. It has been argued from histological evidence that cell-mediated mechanisms of injury are likely to be paramount in clinical TIN[119]. As most of the cells in the interstitium are T-helper cells, delayed hypersensitivity reactions are more likely than direct cytotoxicity. The occasional reports of *in vitro* blast transformation occurring in patients with TIN on exposure of their cells to the initiating drug are of considerable interest and may provide important information on the pathogenesis of the condition[58,83,92].

DIAGNOSIS OF DRUG-INDUCED TIN

A complete history of drug intake (both prescribed and self-administered) and of any possible environmental or occupational toxic exposure must be obtained from any patient with renal failure of obscure aetiology. Details of clinical presentations of TIN induced by individual drugs have been given earlier in this chapter but it is worth stressing that there are at least two main types of presentation. The first is typified by 'methicillin nephritis', occurs several days after regular intake of the drug has commenced and has a rather indolent presentation. This may be contrasted with the more acute, multisystem disturbance, which may follow re-exposure to a drug, such as rifampicin, well tolerated during a previous course of treatment. In such a case, the presentation tends to be sudden, with fever, rigors, arthralgia, nausea, vomiting, diarrhoea and oliguria occurring within hours of rechallenge. Although such features as modest proteinuria (less than 2 g/24 h), glycosuria, haematuria, sterile pyuria, eosinophilia, eosinophiluria, and raised serum IgE levels support a diagnosis of TIN they are not specific and acute TIN may develop in their absence. Renal biopsy is then particularly helpful in confirming a clinically suspected diagnosis or in raising its possibility in a patient with ARF of uncertain origin. Similarly, renal biopsy may help the differentiation between chronic TIN and other renal parenchymal pathology in patients with chronic renal failure and unscarred kidneys.

Radionuclide imaging of the normal kidney with gallium-67 shows that little gallium remains 24 hours after injection. Intense uptake, persisting for 24–72 hours has been claimed as characteristic of acute TIN whether or not caused by drugs. Wood *et al.* reported three such cases[120]. In the first, scanning for suspected occult sepsis showed intense uptake at 24, 48 and 72 hours. Sepsis was not proven, renal biopsy showed florid TIN and the fever and renal abnormalities resolved rapidly with prednisolone treatment. Repeat scanning after 11 days treatment showed no uptake at 24 hours. The cause of the biopsy-proven TIN was uncertain. The second case had SLE with heavy lymphocytic interstitial infiltration as well as a membranous nephropathy. Gallium scanning showed intense renal uptake at 24–48 hours which was reduced after two weeks prednisolone treatment. The third case was dialysis dependent, with focal segmental glomerulonephritis and TIN on biopsy; there was intense renal uptake of gallium 24–72 hours after injection. Linton *et al.*[2] demonstrated similar changes in nine cases of drug-induced biopsy-proven TIN; they were also found in one patient not subjected to renal biopsy who had acute renal failure, haematuria and eosinophilia associated with intravenous cefoxitin treatment[78].

Although the changes on gallium scanning are characteristic, they are not specific for TIN and have also been found in patients with vasculitis or acute pyelonephritis[121] as well as in nephrotic syndrome associated with minimal change glomerulonephritis[2]. These conditions can, however, usually be differentiated from acute TIN on other grounds. Although Kumar and Coleman[121] claimed that abnormal gallium scans occurred in two renal-transplant patients with acute tubular necrosis, biopsies were not performed and the diagnosis, from the data presented, was not secure. In contrast, Linton *et al.*[2] found no renal uptake of gallium in six cases of acute tubular necrosis, although, once more, full clinical details were not given. The intensity of gallium uptake does not, however, correlate with the degree of interstitial infiltration in patients with glomerulonephritis[122].

Gallium may, therefore, be useful in differentiating acute TIN from acute tubular necrosis. Pagniez *et al.*[123] performed gallium scans on 31 patients with acute renal failure of recent onset. In 12 of the 14 with no significant uptake at 48 hours, the renal failure resolved (the presumptive diagnosis being acute tubular necrosis), one patient died and one had bilateral renal artery occlusion. Four of the 14 with persisting bilateral uptake were biopsied and had TIN, the remainder recovering without biopsy. Three had unilateral uptake and were presumed, for this reason, to have unsuspected acute pyelonephritis.

TREATMENT AND PROGNOSIS

In addition to withdrawal of the suspected drug and the usual management of renal failure, steroids, often in high dose, are frequently recommended for the treatment of acute drug-induced TIN. There are numerous case reports detailing a favourable clinical outcome, with rapid resolution of systemic symptoms, such as fever, and the prompt onset of diuresis coincident with steroid therapy[15,25,41,57]. Selective reporting, however, and uncertainty over the natural history of the condition after withdrawal of the causative drug usually makes it impossible to be confident that the steroid treatment was responsible for improvement in an individual patient.

One report attempting to compare the effect of giving prednisolone with that of withholding it in patients with TIN[25], was flawed. Fourteen patients, treated in two different hospitals, were studied. They had developed renal failure, suspected as due to methicillin-induced TIN. The methicillin had been given prophylactically before cardiac surgery (4 patients) or for infection, usually staphylococcal (10 patients). The diagnosis of TIN was supported by fever, eosinophilia and pyuria, without any other apparent cause. Only 8 patients underwent renal biopsy and this confirmed acute TIN in each case. Additional histological changes included mild arteriolitis (2 patients), arteriolar sclerosis (2 patients) and diabetic nephropathy (in 2 known diabetics). The four patients managed in one hospital, and the first two who presented in the other, were treated without prednisolone. The next 8 patients, all from the second hospital, were given an average dose of prednisolone of 60 mg per day for an average of 10 days. Therefore, treatment was not randomized; it was biased according to the treatment centre and steroid therapy was not standardized in dosage or duration. The authors reported that 7 of the 8 who received steroids 'responded promptly with a rapid return to near normal renal function'. In the patients who did not receive prednisolone, 'renal failure persisted longer'. Although the rate of fall in serum creatinine concentration was claimed to be significantly greater in the prednisolone-treated group, 3 patients treated with steroids and 2 in the untreated group required dialysis which makes assessment of the rate of change of serum creatinine uninterpretable. For the same reason, the data presented to show that 'the average number of days from peak serum creatinine to the new baseline' was 9.3 in the patients receiving prednisolone and 54 in those not receiving it, are also unreliable – dialysis would have obscured the time at which serum creatinine peaked. Although the difference was not significant, the final serum creatinine in 6 of 8 patients treated with prednisolone, compared with 2 of the 6 not so treated, was similar to the first recorded concentration. Two of the untreated patients took much longer than the other patients to reach the nadirs in their serum creatinine concentration. Of interest is one patient whose renal function deteriorated after prednisolone treatment was stopped, only to improve markedly when a second course was given.

A more recent report is that of Buysen *et al.*[124] who studied 27 patients with biopsy-proven TIN of drug-induced, infectious or uncertain causation. In 17 patients, renal function improved soon after withdrawal of the drug or treatment of infection. However, in 10 patients, no recovery was observed in the first five days. These were treated with high-dose prednisolone following which the decline in renal function was reversed. The treatment was not randomized; the treated groups were not comparable and the conclusion that steroids were beneficial is not beyond doubt.

Pusey *et al.*[57] compared the progress of 7 patients, treated for biopsy-proven drug-induced TIN with high doses of intravenous methyl prednisolone, with that of 2 patients not given steroids. The causative drugs were co-trimoxazole, ampicillin, ampicillin plus flucloxacillin, penicillin, gentamicin, paracetamol and bendrofluazide. All steroid-treated patients developed a diuresis or a reduction in serum creatinine not attributable to dialysis within 72 hours, and creatinine clearance stabilized between 68 and 90 ml/min. One of the 2 who did not receive steroid therapy recovered normal renal function slowly (final creatinine clearance 82 ml/min) and one was left with a clearance of only 15 ml/min.

A beneficial effect of steroid therapy, even if the sensitizing drug is not withdrawn, is suggested by a single case report[125]. The patient, receiving long-term sulphasalazine for Crohn's disease, was prescribed cimetidine 5 weeks prior to hospital admission, when serum creatinine was 280 μmol/l and there was eosinophilia, sterile pyuria and a trace of proteinuria. After sulphasalazine had been stopped, cimetidine was continued, and serum creatinine increased, necessitating haemodialysis. Renal biopsy revealed acute TIN and prednisolone (80 mg per day) appeared to cause a rapid reduction in serum creatinine to 240 μmol/l. When the prednisolone dosage was reduced, serum creatinine rose again to 380 μmol/l. After cimetidine had been stopped and the steroids temporarily increased, there was 'a dramatic improvement in renal function'.

There is at least one case report suggesting that steroid treatment may improve TIN which is deteriorating despite withdrawal of the causative agent. Robson *et al.*[38] reported acute renal failure complicating sulphadiazine treatment of urinary tract infection. The drug was stopped after 9 days and renal biopsy showed interstitial oedema and infiltration with numerous polymorphonuclear leucocytes and a few eosinophils; no sulphonamide crystals were seen. The patient was virtually anuric and dialysis dependent for a further 5 weeks. Repeat biopsy 26 days after cessation of sulphadiazine showed even more severe interstitial changes. Prednisolone (40 mg per day) was administered, diuresis occurred within 24 hours and the patient became dialysis independent. Four months after stopping sulphadiazine, the patient's creatinine clearance was 65 ml/min and a third renal biopsy showed marked interstitial fibrosis and tubular atrophy. Skin patch tests for sulphadiazine allergy were negative.

In another case report[126] of a patient with biopsy-proven acute TIN of uncertain origin, the administration of prednisolone after 3 months of regular dialysis appeared to improve renal function, the final serum creatinine concentration falling to 180 μmol/l.

Thus although the value of steroid treatment in acute drug-induced TIN has not been proved scientifically, a number of case reports suggest that prednisolone in doses of 40–60 mg per day improves renal function – perhaps even in patients requiring dialysis treatment. The prognosis for recovery of renal function after TIN is, in general, good, but there may be significant residual impairment and chronic interstitial fibrosis may sometimes develop within a few weeks.

REFERENCES

1. Hansen, H. E. and Amdisen, A. (1978). Lithium intoxication. Report of 23 cases and review of 100 cases from the literature. *Q. J. Med.*, **47**, 123–144

2. Linton, A. L., Clark, W. F., Driedgar, A. A., Turnbull, D. R. and Lindsey, R. M. (1980). Acute interstitial nephritis due to drugs. *Ann. Int. Med.*, **93,** 735–741
3. Kleinknecht, D., Vanhille, Ph., Morel-Maroger, L., Kanfer, A., Lemaitre, V., Mery, J. P., Laederich, L. and Callard, P. (1983). Acute interstitial nephritis due to drug hypersensitivity. An up to date review with a report of 19 cases. *Adv. Nephrol.*, **12,** 277–308
4. Richet, G., Sraer, J. D., Kowilsy, O., Kanfer, A., Mignon, F., Whitworth, J., Morel-Morages, L. *et al.* (1978), La production biopsie rénale dans l'insuffisance rénale aigue. *Ann. Med. Interne*, **129,** 445–447
5. Grunfeld, J. P., Kleinknecht, D. and Droz, D. (1988). Acute interstitial nephritis. In Schries, R. W. and Gottschalk, C. W. (eds). *Diseases of the Kidney*, Vol. II, 4th Edn., pp. 1462–1463. (Boston/Toronto: Little, Brown and Co.)
6. Wilson, D. M., Turner, D. R., Cameron, J. S., Ogg, C. S., Brown, C. B. and Chantler, C. (1976). Value of renal biopsy in acute intrinsic renal failure. *Br. Med. J.*, **2,** 459–461
7. Sarjad, S. A., Haddad, G. G. and Nassar, V. H. (1974). Nephropathy, as underestimated complication of methicillin therapy. *J Paediatr.*, **84,** 873–877
8. Nolan, C. M. and Abernathy, R. S. (1977). Nephropathy associated with methicillin therapy. *Arch. Intern. Med.*, **137,** 997–1000
9. Appel, G. B. and Neu, H. G. (1984). Acute interstitial nephritis induced by *β* lactam antibiotics. In Fillastre, J. H., Whelton, A. and Tulkens, P (eds.) *Antibiotic Nephrotoxicity*. (Paris: INSERM)
10. Baldwin, D. S., Levine, B. B., McCluskey, R. T. and Gallo, G. R. (1968). Renal failure and interstitial nephritis due to penicillin and methicillin. *N. Engl. J. Med.* **279,** 1245–1252
11. Becq-Giraudon, B., Talin D'Eyzac, A., Reboux, J. F., Alcalay, D. and Sudre, Y. (1974). Les nephropathies de la methicilline. *Nouv. Presse Méd.*, **3,** 2509
12. Border, W. A., Lehman, D. H., Egan, J. D., Sass, H. J., Glode, J. E. and Wilson, C. B. (1974). Antitubular basement membrane antibodies in methicillin-associated interstitial nephritis. *N. Engl. J. Med.*, **291,** 381–384
13. Ditlove, J., Weidmann, P., Bernstein, M. and Massry, S. G. (1977). Methicillin nephritis. *Medicine* (*Baltimore*), **56,** 483–491
14. Maynaud, C., Kanfer, A., Kourilsky, O. and Straer, J. D. (1975). Interstitial nephritis after methicillin. *N. Engl. J. Med.*, **292,** 1132—1133
15. Gilbert, D. N., Gourley, R., d'Agostino, A., Goodnight, S. H. Jr and Worthen, H. (1970). Interstitial nephritis due to methicillin, penicillin and ampicillin. *Ann. Allergy*, **28,** 378–385
16. Hansen, E. S. and Tauris, P. (1976). Methicillin-induced nephropathy. *Acta Pathol. Microbiol. Scand.*, **84,** 440–442
17. Hewitt, W. L., Finegold, S. M. and Monzon, O. T. (1961). Untoward side effects associated with methicillin therapy. *Antimicrob. Agents Chemother.*, **1,** 765–769
18. London, R. D. (1967). Haematuria associated with methicillin therapy. *J. Paediatr.*, **70,** 285–286
19. Mayaud, C., Kanfer, A., Kourilsky, O. and Straer, J. D. (1975). Interstitial nephritis after methicillin. *N. Engl. J. Med.*, **292,** 1132–1133
20. Minetti, L., Barbiano di Belgiojoso, G., Civati, G., Durante, A., Ratti, F. and Rovati, C. (1974). Nefiti da ipersensibilità a farmaci (NIF): Osservazioni clinicoistologiche in 15 anni. *Minerva Nefrol.*, **21,** 197–212
21. Olsen, S. and Asklund, M. (1976). Interstitial nephritis with acute renal failure

following cardiac surgery and treatment with methicillin. *Acta Med. Scand.*, **199,** 305–310
22. Ooi, B. S, Pesce, A. J, First, M. R., Pollak, V. E., Bernstein, I. L. and Jao, W. (1974). IgE levels in interstitial nephritis. *Lancet*, **1,** 1254–1256
23. Simenhoff, M. L., Guild, W. R. and Dammin, G. J. (1968). Acute diffuse interstitial nephritis. *Am. J. Med.*, **44,** 618–625
24. Woodroffe, A. J., Thomson, N. M., Meadows, R. and Lawrence, J. R. (1974). Nephropathy associated with methicillin administration. *Aust. NZ J. Med.*, **4,** 256–261
25. Galpin, J. E., Shinaberger, J. H., Stanley, T. M., Blumenkrantz, M. J., Bayer, A. S., Friedman, G. S., Montogomerie, J. Z., Guze, L. B., Coburn, J. W. and Glassock, R. J. (1978). Acute interstitial nephritis due to methicillin. *Am. J. Med.*, **65,** 756–765
26. Woodroffe, A. J., Thomson, N. M., Meadows, S. R. and Lawrence, J. R. (1974). Nephropathy associated with methicillin administration. *Aust. NZ J. Med.*, **4,** 256–261
27. Gilbert, D. M., Gourley, R., D'Argostino, A., Goodnight, S. H. Jnr., Worthen, H. (1970). Interstitial nephritis due to methicillin, penicillin and ampicillin. *Ann. Allergy.*, **28,** 378–385
28. Appel, G. B. and Neu, H. C. (1977). The nephrotoxicity of antimicrobial agents. *N. Engl. J. Med.*, **296,** 663–670
29. French, A. J. (1946). Hypersensitivity in the pathogenesis of the histopathologic changes associated with sulphonamide chemotherapy. *Am. J. Pathol.*, **22,** 679–701
30. More, R. H., McMillan, G. C. and Duff, G. L. (1946). The pathology of sulphonamide allergy in man. *Am. J. Pathol.*, **22,** 703–735
31. Fuller, T. J., Barcenas, G.C. and White, M. G. (1976). Diuretic induced interstitial nephritis. Occurrence in a patient with membranous glomerulonephritis. *J. Am. Med. Assoc.*, **235,** 1998–1999.
32. Magil, A. B., Ballon, A. B. and Cameron, E. C. (1980). Acute interstitial nephritis associated with thiazide diuretics. Clinical and pathological observation in three cases. *Am. J. Med.*, **69,** 939
33. Nessi, R., Bonoldi, G. L., Redaelli, B. and DiFillippo, G. (1976). Acute renal failure after rifampicin. A case report and survey of the literature. *Nephron*, **16,** 148–159
34. Rothwell, D. L. and Richmond, D. E. (1971). Hepatorenal failure with self-initiated intermittent rifampicin therapy. *Br. Med. J.*, **12,** 491
35. Straer, J. D., Beaufils, P., Morel-Maroger, L. and Richet, G. (1972). Nephrite interstitielle chronique due a la phenylindanedione faisant suite à une insuffisance rénale aigue. *Nouv. Presse Méd.*, **1,** 193–196
36. Cogan, M. C. and Arieff, A. L. (1978). Sodium wasting, acidosis and hyperkalemia induced by methicillin interstitial nephritis. Evidence for selective distal tubular dysfunction. *Am. J. Med.*, **65,** 756
37. Appel, G. B. and Kumis, C. L. (1982). Acute tubulointerstitial nephritis. In Cotran, R. S. (ed.) *Tubulointerstitial Nephropathies. Contemporary issues in Nephrology*, Vol. 10, pp. 151–186. (New York: Churchill Livingstone)
38. Robson, M., Leri, J., Dolberg, L. and Rosenfeld, J. B. (1970). Acute tubulointerstitial nephritis following sulphadiazine therapy. *Israel J. Med. Sci.*, **61,** 561–566

39. Burghard, R., Brandis, M. and Hoyer, P. F. (1984). Acute interstitial nephritis in childhood. *Eur. J. Paediatr.*, **142,** 103
40. Dry, J., Leynadier, F., Herman, D. and Pradalier, A. (1975). L'association sulfamethoxazole-trimethoprime (cotrimoxazole). Reaction immuno-allergique inhabituelle. *Nouv. Presse Méd.*, **4,** 36
41. Kalowski, S., Nanra, R. S., Matthew, T. H. and Kincaid-Smith, P. (1973). Deterioration in renal function in association with cotrimoxazole therapy. *Lancet*, **1,** 394–397
42. Flynn, C. T., Rainford, D. J. and Hope, E. (1974). Acute renal failure and rifampicin: Danger of unsuspected intermittent dosage. *Br. Med. J.*, **2,** 482
43. Cordonnier, D. and Muller, J. M. (1972). Acute renal failure after rifampicin. *Lancet*, **2,** 1364–1365
44. Kleinknecht, D., Homberg, J. C. and Decroix, G. (1972). Acute renal failure after rifampicin. *Lancet*, **1,** 1238–1239
45. Poole, G., Stradling, P. and Worlledge, S. (1971). Potentially serious side-effects of high dose twice weekly rifampicin. *Br. Med. J.*, **3,** 343–347
46. Ramgopal, V., Leonard, C. and Bhathena, D. (1973). Acute renal failure associated with rifampicin. *Lancet*, **1,** 1195–1196
47. Qunibi, Y. W., Godwin, J. and Eknoyan, G. (1980). Toxic nephropathy during continuous rifampicin therapy. *South. Med. J.*, **73,** 791–792
48. Bansal, V. K., Bennett, B. and Molnar, Z. (1977). Prolonged renal failure after rifampicin. *Am. Rev. Respir. Dis.*, **116,** 137–140
49. Kleinknecht, D., Homberg, J. C. and Decroix, G. (1972). Acute renal failure after rifampicin. *Lancet*, **1,** 1238–1239
50. Cochran, M., Moorhead, P. J. and Platts, M. (1975). Permanent renal damage with rifampicin. *Lancet*, **1,** 1428
51. Conen, D., Blumberg, A., Weber, S. and Schubothe, H. (1979). Hamolytische krise und akutes nierenversagenunter rifampicin. *Schweiz Med. Wochenschr.*, **109,** 558–562
52. Kleinknecht, D., Kanfer, A. and Mori-Aroger, L. (1978). Immunologically mediated drug induced acute renal failure. In *Contributions in Nephrology*, Vol. 10, p. 42. (Basel: S. Karger)
53 Mery, J Ph and Morel-Morager, L. (1976). Les nephrites interstitielles aigue par hypersensibilite medicamenteuse. *Ann. Med. Interne*, **127,** 590–595
54. Straer, J. D., Beaufils, P., Morel-Maroger, L. and Richet, G. (1972). Nephrite interstitielle chronique due a la phenylindanedione faisant suite a une insuffisance rénale aigue. *Nouv. Presse Méd.*, **1,** 193–196
55. Peskow, S. T., McMillan, J. R., Lorch, A., Sussman, H. and Ozava, T. (1978). Reversible acute renal failure associated with chlorthalidone therapy: possible drug induced interstitial nephritis. *J. Med. Assoc. George*, **67,** 17–18
56. Magil, A. B. (1983). Drug induced acute interstitial nephritis with granulomas. *Hum. Pathol.*, **13,** 36
57. Pusey, C. D., Saltiss, D., Bloodworth, L., Rainford, D. J. and Christie, J. L. (1983). Drug associated acute interstitial nephritis: Clinical and pathological features and the response to high dose steroid therapy. *Q. J. Med.*, **206,** 194–211
58. Bailey, R. R., Lynn, K. L. and Drennan, C. J. (1982). Triamterene induced acute interstitial nephritis. *Lancet*, **1,** 226
59. Fuller, T. J., Barcenas, C. G. and White, M. G. (1976). Diuretic induced interstitial nephritis. *J. Am. Med. Assoc.*, **235,** 1998–1999

60. Chevet, D., Pogamp, P., Guivarch, G. *et al.* (1983). Nephrites interstitielles aigues induites par triamterene et thiazides. *Nephrologie*, **4,** 38
61. Fialk, M. A., Romankiewicz, J., Perrone, F. and Sherman, R. L. (1974). Allergic interstitial nephritis with diuretics. *Ann. Intern. Med.*, **81,** 403–404
62. Colvin, R. B., Burton, J. R., Hyslop, N. E. Jr., Spitz, L. and Lichenstein, N. S. (1974). Penicillin associated interstitial nephritis. *Ann. Intern. Med.*, **81,** 404–405
63. Ruley, E. J. and Lisi, L. M. (1974). Interstitial nephritis and renal failure due to ampicillin. *J. Paediatr.*, **84,** 878–881
64. Tannenberg, A. M., Wicher, K. J. and Rose, N. R. (1971). Ampicillin nephropathy. *J. Am. Med. Assoc.*, **218,** 449
65. Maxwell, D., Szwed, J. J., Wahle, W. and Kleit, S. A. (1974). Ampicillin nephropathy. *J. Am. Med. Assoc.*, **230,** 586–587
66. Appe, G. B., Garvey, G., Silva, F., Franke, E., Neu, H. C. and Weissman, J. (1981). Acute interstitial nephritis due to amoxycillin therapy. *Nephron*, **27,** 313–315
67. Burton, J. R., Lichenstein, N. S., Colvin, R. B. and Hyslop, N. E. Jr. (1974). Acute interstitial nephritis from oxacillin. *Johns Hopkins Med. J.*, **134,** 58–61
68. Tillman, D. B., Oill, P. A. and Guze, L. B. (1980). Oxacillin nephritis. *Arch. Intern. Med.*, **140,** 1552
69. Parry, M. F., Ball, W. D., Contre, J. E. Jr and Cohen, S. N. (1973). Nafcillin-nephritis. *J. Am. Med. Assoc.*, **225,** 178
70. Appel, G. B., Woda, B. A., Neu, H. C., Parry, M. F., Silva, F. and Pirani, C. L. (1978). Acute interstitial nephritis associated with carbenicillin therapy. *Arch. Intern. Med.*, **138,** 1265–1267
71. Roselle, G. A., Glyne, D. H. and Kauffman, C. A. (1978). Carbenicillin nephrotoxicity. *South. Med. J.*, **71,** 84–86
72. Durham, D. S. and Ibels, L. S. (1981). Cephalothin induced acute allergic interstitial nephritis. *Aust. NZ J. Med.*, **11,** 266–267
73. Verma, S. and Kieff, E. (1975). Cephalexin related nephropathy. *J. Am. Med. Assoc.*, **234,** 618–619
74. Millman, M. (1946). Acute interstitial nephritis during treatment with penicillin and cephalothin. *Acta Med. Scand.*, **203,** 227–230
75. Wiles, C. M., Assem, S. K., Cohen, S. L. and Fisher, C. (1979). Cephradine induced interstitial nephritis. *Clin. Exp. Immunol.*, **36,** 342–346
76. Engle, J. E., Drago, J., Carlin, B. and Schoolworth, A. C. (1975). Reversible acute renal failure after cephalothin. *Ann. Intern. Med.*, **83,** 232–233
77. Appel, G. B. and Kunis, C. L. (1983). Acute tubulointerstitial nephritis. In R. S. Cotran, B. M. Brenner and J. H. Stein (eds.) *Tubulointerstitial Nephropathies*, pp. 151–185. (New York: Churchill)
78. Haskell, R. J., Fujita, N. K., Stevenson, J. A. and Border, W. A. (1981). Cefoxitin induced interstitial nephritis. *Arch. Intern. Med.*, **141,** 1557
79. Hestbech, H., Hansen, H. E., Amdisen, A. and Olsen, O. (1977). Chronic renal lesions following longterm treatment with lithium. *Kidney Int.*, **12,** 205–213
80. Hansen, H. E., Hestbech, J., Sotensen, J. L., Norgaard, K., Heilskov, J. and Amdisen, A. (1979). Chronic interstitial nephropathy in patients on longterm lithium treatment. *Q. J. Med.*, NS **48,** 577–591
81. Bucht, G. and Wahlin, A. (1980). Renal concentrating capacity after longterm lithium treatment and after withdrawal of lithium. *Acta Med. Scand.*, **207,** 309–314

82. Kincaid-Smith, P., Burrows, G. D., Davies, B. M., Holwil, B., Walter, M. and Walker, R. G. (1979). Renal biopsy findings in lithium and pre-lithium patients. *Lancet*, **2,** 700–701
83. Hyman, L. R., Ballow, M. and Kneiser, M. R. (1978). Diphenylhydantoin interstitial nephritis. Roles of cellular and humoral immunologic injury. *J. Pediatr.*, **92,** 915–920
84. Sheth, K. J., Casper, J. T. and Good, T. A. (1977). Interstitial nephritis due to phenytoin hypersensitivity. *J. Pediatr.*, **91,** 438–441
85. Ooi, B. S., Ooi, Y. M., Mohini, R. and Pollak, V. E. (1978). Humoral mechanisms in drug-induced acute interstitial nephritis. *Clin. Immunol. Immunopathol.*, **10,** 330–334
86. Young, J. L., Boswell, R. B and Nils, A. S. (1974). Severe allopurinol hypersensitivity. *Arch. Intern. Med.*, **134,** 553–558
87. Mills, R. M. (1971). Severe hypersensitivity reactions associated with allopurinol. *J. Am. Med. Assoc.*, **216,** 799–802
88. Gelbert, D. R., Weinstein, A. B. and Fajardo, L. F. (1977). Allopurinol induced interstitial nephritis. *Ann. Int. Med.*, **86,** 196–198
89. McKendrick, M. W. and Geddes, A. M. (1979). Allopurinol hypersensitivity. *Br. Med. J.*, **1,** 988
90. McGowen, W. R. and Vermillion, S. E. (1980). Acute interstitial nephritis related to cimetidine therapy. *Gastroenterology*, **79,** 746–749
91. Hake, D. D. (1981). Interstitial nephritis and cimetidine. *Ann. Intern. Med.*, **94,** 416
92. Watson, A. J. S., Dalbow, M. H., Strachura, I., Fragola, J. A., Rubin, M. F., Watson, R. M. and Bourke, E. (1983). Immunologic studies in cimetidine induced nephropathy and polymyositis. *N. Engl. J. Med.*, **308,** 142–145
93. Richman, A. L., Narrajan, J. L. and Hirschfield, J. S. (1981). Acute interstitial nephritis and acute renal failure associated with cimetidine therapy. *Am. J. Med.*, **70,** 1272–1274
94. Dentino, M., Luft, R. C., Yum, N. M., Williams, D. S. and Einhorn, L. H. (1972). Longterm effect of *cis*-diamminedichloroplatinum(II) (NSC119875, CACP). *Cancer*, **30,** 1451
95. Rossof, A. J., Slayton, R. E. and Perlia, C. P. (1972). Preliminary clinical experience with *cis*-diamminedichloroplatinum(II) (NSC119875, CACP). *Cancer*, **30,** 1451
96. Gonzalez-Vitale, J. C., Hayes, D. M., Cvitkovic, E. and Steinberg, S. (1977). The renal pathology in clinical trials of *cis*-platinum(II) diamminedichloride. *Cancer*, **39,** 1362
97. McClusky, R. T. and Colvin, R.-B. (1978). Immunological aspects of renal tubular and interstitial diseases. *Ann. Rev. Med.*, **29,** 191–203
98. Unanue, E. R., Dixon, F. J. and Feldman, J. D. (1967). Experimental allergic glomerulonephritis induced in the rabbit with homologous renal antigens. *J. Exp. Med.*, **125,** 163–176
99. Klassen, J., McClusky, R. T. and Milgrom, F. (1971). Nonglomerular renal disease produced in rabbits by immunization with homologous kidney. *Am. J. Pathol.*, **63,** 333–358
100. Brentjohns, J. R., O'Connell, D. W., Pawlowski, B. and Andres, G. A. (1974). Extraglomerular lesions associated with deposition of circulating antigen–anti-

body couplers in kidneys of rabbits with chronic serum sickness. *Int. Immunol. Immunopathol.*, **3,** 112–118

101. Patrick, C. C., Virella, G., McManus, J. F. A., Faulk, W. P., Hughson, H. D. and Fundenberg, H. H. (1979). Induction of extra-glomerular renal damage in experimental chronic serum sickness. 1. Histologic and immunofluorescence findings. *Lab. Invest.*, **40,** 603–614.
102. Hoyer, J. R. (1980). Tubulointerstitial immune complex nephritis in rats immunized with Tamm-Horsfall protein. *Kidney Int.*, **17,** 284–292
103. Hoyer, J. R. and Seiler, M. W. (1979). Pathophysiology of Tamm-Horsfall protein. *Kidney Int.*, **16,** 279–289
104. Friedman, J., Hoyer, J. R. and Seiler, M. W. (1982). Formation and clearance of tubulointerstitial immune complexes in kidneys of rats immunized with heterologous antisera to Tamm-Horsfall protein. *Kidney Int.*, **21,** 575–582
105. Brentjons, J. R., Sopulveda, M., Baliah, T., Bentzel, C, Erlanger, B. F., Elwood, C., Montes, M., Hsu, K. C. and Andres, G. A. (1975). Interstitial immune complex nephritis in patients with systemic lupus erythematosus. *Kidney Int.*, **7,** 342–350
106. Park, M. H., D'Agati, V., Appel, G. B. and Pirani, C. L. (1986). Tubulointerstitial disease in lupus nephritis: relationship to immune deposits, interstitial inflammation, glomerular changes, renal function and progression. *Nephron*, **44,** 309–319
107. Hyun, J. and Galen, M. A. (1987). Acute interstitial nephritis – a case characterised by increase in serum IgG, IgM and IgE concentrations, eosinophilia and IgE deposition in renal tubules. *Arch. Intern. Med.*, **141,** 679–687
108. Spital, A., Panner, B. J., Stern, R. H. (1987). Primary acute idiopathic tubulointerstitial nephritis: report of two cases and review of the literature. *Am. J. Kidney Dis.*, **9,** 710–718
109. Steblay, R. W. and Rudofsky, U. (1971). Renal tubular disease and autoantibodies against tubular basement membrane induced in guinea pigs. *J. Immunol.*, **107,** 589–594
110. Lehman, D. H., Marquardt, H., Wilson, C. B. and Dixon, F. J. (1974). Specificity of autoantibodies in tubular and glomerular basement membranes induced in guinea pigs. *J. Immumol.*, **112,** 241–248
111. Sugusaki, T., Klassen, J., Milgrom, F., Andres, G. A. and McClusky, R. T. (1973). Immunopathologic study of an autoimmune tubular and interstitial renal disease in Brown Norway rats. *Lab. Invest.*, **28,** 658–671
112. Lehman, D. H., Wilson, C. B. and Dixon, F. J. (1974). Interstitial nephritis in rats immunized with heterologous tubular basement membrane. *Kidney Int.*, **5,** 187–195
113. Rudofsky, U. H., Steblay, R. W. and Pollara, B. (1975). Inhibition of experimental autoimmune renal tubulointerstitial disease in guinea pigs by depletion of complement with cobra venom factor. *Clin. Immunopathol.*, **3,** 396–407
114. Rudofsky, U., McMaster, P. R. B., Ma, W. S., Steblay, R. W. and Pollara, B. (1974). Experimental autoimmune renal cortical tubulointerstitial disease in guinea pigs lacking the fourth component of complement (C4). *J. Immunol.*, **112,** 1387–1393
115. Rudofsky, U. H. and Pollara, B. (1976). Studies of the pathogenesis of experimental autoimmune renal tubulointerstitial disease in guinea pigs. *Clin. Immunol. Immunopathol.*, **6,** 107–114

116. Van Zweiten, M. J., Leber, P. D., Bhan, A. K. and McClusky, R. T. (1977). Experimental cell mediated interstitial nephritis induced with exogenous antigens. *J. Immunol.*, **118,** 589–593
117. Baldamas, C. A., Kachel, G., Koch, C. and Schoeppe, W. (1979). Cellular immune mechanisms in experimental tubulointerstitial nephritis (TIN). *Contr. Nephrol.*, **16,** 141
118. Kelly, C. J., Korngold, R., Mann, R., Clayman, M., Haverty, T. and Neilson, E. G. (1986). Spontaneous interstitial nephritis in kdkd mice 11. Characterisation of a tubular antigen specific H-2-K restricted Lyt 2 D+ effector cell that mediates destructive tubulointerstitial injury. *J. Immunol.*, **136,** 536–531
119. Cameron, J. S. (1988). Allergic interstitial nephritis: Clinical features and pathogenesis. *Q. J. Med.*, **66,** 97–115
120. Wood, B. C., Sharma, J. N., Germann, D. R., Wood, W. G. and Crouch, T. T. (1978). Gallium citrate 67 imaging in non-infectious interstitial nephritis. *Arch. Int. Med.*, **138,** 1665–1666
121. Kumar, B. and Coleman, R. E. (1976). Significance of delayed 67Ga localisation in kidneys. *J. Nucl. Med.*, **17,** 872–875
122. Moulin, B., Sahali, D., Baud, L., Toussaint, P., Michel, C., Ronco, P. and Mignon, F. (1988). Gallium 67 scintigraphy in the diagnosis of glomerulonephritis. *Clin. Nephrol.*, **30,** 128–133
123. Pagniez, D., Beauscat, L., Delvallez, P., Dequidt, P. and Tacquet, A. (1988). Renal gallium scan in acute renal failure. *Nephrodial. Transplant.*, **3,4,** 535
124. Buysen, J. G. M., Krediet, R. T. and Arisz, L. (1988). Acute interstitial nephritis. Clinical presentation and effect of treatment with corticosteroids. *Nephrol. Dial. Transplant.*, **3,4,** 507
125. Richman, A. V., Narayan, J. L. and Hirschfield, J. S. (1981). Acute interstitial nephritis and acute renal failure associated with cimetidine. *Am. J. Med.*, **70,** 1272
126. Frommer, P., Uldall, R., Fag, W. P. and Deveber, G. A. (1979). A case of acute interstitial nephritis fully treated after delayed diagnosis. *Can Med. Assoc. J.*, **121,** 585–586
127. Luderer, J. R., Schoolworth, A. C., Sinicrope, R. A., Ballard, J. O., Lokingbill, D. P. and Hayes, A. H. (1981). Acute renal failure, haemolytic anaemia and skin rash associated with captopril therapy. *Am. J. Med.*, **71,** 493–496
128. Hogg, R. J., Sawyer, M. and Hecox, K. (1981). Carbamazepine induced acute tubulointerstitial nephritis. *J. Paediatr.*, **98,** 830
129. Cumming, A. (1980). Acute renal failure and interstitial nephritis after clofibrate treatment. *Br. Med. J.*, **281,** 1529–1530
130. Averbuch, S. D., Austen, H. A., Sherwin, S. A., Antonorych, T., Bunn, P. A. and Longo, D. L. (1984). Acute interstitial nephritis with the nephrotic syndrome following recombinant leukocyte A interferon therapy for mycosis fungoides. *N. Engl. J. Med.*, **310,** 32–35
131. Walker, R. G., Thomson, N. M., Dowling, J. P. and Ogg, C. S. (1979). Minocycline induced acute interstitial nephritis. *Br. Med. J.*, **1,** 524
132. Ihle, B. U., Byrnes, C. A. and Simenhoff, M. L. (1982). Acute renal failure due to interstitial nephritis resulting from radio-contrast agents. *Aust. NZ J. Med.*, **12,** 630–632
133. Walker, R. G., Whitworth, J. A. and Kincaid-Smith, P. (1980). Acute interstitial nephritis in a patient taking tienilic acid. *Br. Med. J.*, **280,** ·1212

134. Eisenberg, E. S., Robbins, N. and Lenci, M. (1981). Vancomycin and interstitial nephritis. *Ann. Intern. Med.*, **95,** 658
135. Rosenfield, J., Gara, V., Boner, G., Ben-Bassat, B. and Lirni, E. (1983). Interstitial nephritis with ARF after erythromycin. *Br. Med. J.*, **286,** 938–939

3

METHODS TO INCREASE POISON ELIMINATION

J. A. VALE

Most poisoned patients recover, at least physically, with little more than nursing care, though about 10% of patients need intensive supportive therapy to maintain vital functions. Methods to increase the elimination of poisons are appropriate in fewer than 5% of cases. Moreover, such techniques should only be undertaken by those experienced in their use as the morbidity and even mortality are otherwise likely to be higher than with supportive measures alone. Yet, as Prescott[1] has argued, 'poisoned patients are often subjected to unnecessary and potentially harmful haemodialysis and forced diuresis. Unfortunately, there are few instances in which these measures have clearly been shown to reduce morbidity and mortality, and much of the information on which claims for efficacy have been based is either inadequate or invalid.... Clinicians seem to have an irresistible urge to carry out some form of treatment on their patients, and this is particularly so for the unconscious patient whose relatives may be clamouring for something to be done. In practice, there are few indications for the use of haemodialysis or forced diuresis to accelerate the removal of drugs in poisoned patients'. This latter statement would also apply to the use of haemoperfusion.

There are four techniques currently available to increase poison elimination:

(1) Forced (alkaline, acid) diuresis;
(2) Repeat-dose activated charcoal therapy;

(3) Dialysis;
(4) Haemoperfusion.

To be valuable clinically, the rate of toxin removal by any of these elimination techniques must be significantly greater than spontaneous rates of elimination by hepatic metabolism or renal excretion.

FORCED DIURESIS

Excretion of Poisons

The filtrate produced by the glomeruli has a composition similar to that of plasma water but excludes molecules with a molecular weight of more than 66 000 Da (which includes drug–protein complexes). Thus, only that fraction of the drug which is free (non-protein-bound) is filtered.

Some drugs are actively secreted into the proximal renal tubules against the concentration gradient. These include acidic drugs, such as the penicillins, sulphonamides, phenobarbitone, salicylates, phenylbutazone and probenecid, and organic bases, such as quinine, quinidine, amphetamine and procainamide.

Drugs may also be eliminated by passive diffusion across the epithelium of the tubule into the lumen. As water is progressively reabsorbed from the tubular fluid as it passes distally, a favourable concentration gradient is created for the reabsorption of these dissolved substances back into the blood stream.

Tubular reabsorption is influenced by urinary flow rate. Diuresis therefore increases renal clearance of drugs that are passively reabsorbed since the concentration gradient is reduced. Potentially, therefore, drugs excreted largely unchanged by the kidney may be removed in significant quantities by increasing urinary flow.

Indications

Forced diuresis has been advocated for the treatment of phenobarbitone, phenytoin and lithium poisoning.

Phenobarbitone

Prescott[1] demonstrated that the clearance of phenobarbitone is directly related to urine flow. The use of forced (alkaline) diuresis in three patients increased the mean clearance of phenobarbitone from 1.8 to 14 ml/min and the maximum excretion rate achieved was 121.2 mg/h. However, these clearance values are very inferior to those obtained by repeat-dose activated charcoal therapy and haemoperfusion. The use of forced diuresis, with or without pH manipulation, in the treatment of phenobarbitone poisoning should therefore be abandoned.

Phenytoin

Although there is experimental evidence[2] that phenytoin clearance may be increased from 5 to 20 ml/min, this is less impressive than the values achieved by body clearance alone[3]. Forced diuresis therefore, has no role in the management of phenytoin overdose.

Lithium

Sodium chloride diuresis has been proposed as a useful means of increasing lithium excretion in intoxicated patients[4]. However, Hansen and Amdisen[5] were unable to demonstrate any specific effect of sodium on lithium excretion since the fractional excretion of lithium did not change consistently during the sodium infusion. This is not surprising, as many of their patients had impaired renal function due to lithium toxicity. Similarly, Jacobsen *et al.*[6] found that forced diuresis with sodium chloride did not significantly increase renal elimination. In contrast, Dyson *et al.*[7] have reported that renal lithium clearance is enhanced by increased sodium excretion.

Although the precise role of forced diuresis in lithium intoxication has not been established, it is probable that forced diuresis with 0.9% sodium chloride may be helpful in patients with normal renal function who are only mildly intoxicated and whose serum lithium con-

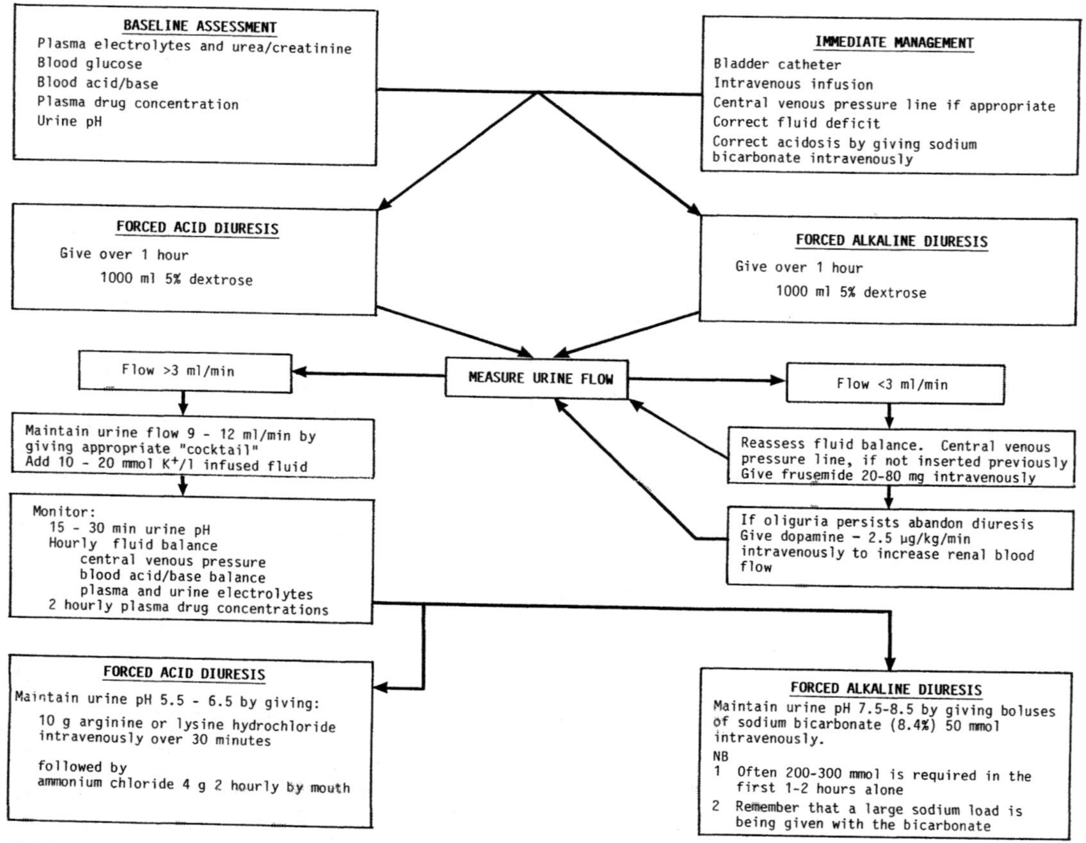

FIGURE 3.1 Procedure for alkaline and acid diuresis in adults

centration does not exceed 3 mmol/l. More severely poisoned patients require haemodialysis.

Large infusions of sodium should be avoided in patients suffering from lithium intoxication because of the risk of producing hypernatraemia due to water-losing nephritis.

Recently, Macdonald *et al.* have advocated[8] the use of low-dose dopamine in lithium intoxication on the basis that dopamine increases sodium excretion by a specific action on the proximal tubule. Further studies are required to confirm this single case observation.

FORCED DIURESIS WITH pH MANIPULATION

Rationale

Most drugs are weak electrolytes which, at physiological pH, exist partly as undissociated molecules. The extent of ionization is a function of the ionization constant (Ka) of the drug and the pH of the medium in which it is dissolved. Ionization constants are expressed in the form of their negative logarithms, pKa. Hence, the stronger an acid, the lower its pKa, and, the stronger a base, the higher the pKa. The relationship between pKa and the proportion of total drug in ionized form is represented by the Henderson–Hasselbach equation:

$$\text{For weak acids, } \mathrm{pH} - \mathrm{pKa} = \log \frac{\text{(ionized drug)}}{\text{(non-ionized drug)}}$$

$$\text{For weak bases, } \mathrm{pH} - \mathrm{pKa} = \log \frac{\text{(non-ionized drug)}}{\text{(ionized drug)}}$$

Thus, when pKa = pH, the concentrations of ionized and non-ionized drug are equal.

Cell membranes are more permeable to substances that are lipid soluble and in the non-ionized, rather than the ionized, form. Thus, the rate of diffusion from the renal tubular lumen back into the circulation is decreased when a drug is maximally ionized. Because ionization of weak acids is increased in an alkaline environment, and that of basic drugs in an acid solution, manipulation of the urinary pH can enhance renal excretion. For acidic drugs, there is a greater degree of ionization at pH 8 than 7.4 and, for basic drugs, a greater degree of ionization at pH 6 than at 7.4. Thus, elimination of weak acids by the kidneys is increased in alkaline urine if the pKa of the drug concerned lies in the range 3.0 to 7.4; for weak bases, elimination is increased in acid urine if the pKa of the drug lies in the range 7.5 to 10.5.

Since pKa is a logarithmic function then, theoretically, a small change in urine pKa could have a disproportionate effect on clearance, especially for those drugs which have pKa values close to blood pH. Thus, the elimination of salicylate (pKa 3.5) is increased in alkaline urine and urinary acidification will increase the elimination of amphetamines (pKa 9.8). If urine pH is decreased to pH 5.5, the elimination of amphetamine is increased some seven times compared with its elimination in individuals with uncontrolled urinary pH (see below).

Use of forced diuresis with pH manipulation is therefore appropriate if:

(1) A substantial proportion of the poison is excreted in the urine in unchanged (i.e. non-metabolized) form or the metabolites themselves are toxic.
(2) The poison is distributed mainly in the extracellular fluid, i.e. the volume of distribution is small.
(3) The poison is minimally protein bound.
(4) Manipulation of urinary pH will maximally ionize the poison, so enhancing elimination.

Procedure – alkaline diuresis

Forced alkaline diuresis has been employed in the management of salicylate poisoning for the last two decades.[9–12] It is now recognized, however, that the urinary pH is of far greater importance than the volume of urine excreted[13,14]. To achieve maximum excretion of salicylate, a urine pH above 7.5, ideally between 8.0 and 8.5, is necessary. Rather than using a standard 'cocktail' as recommended by Lawson *et al.*[12], the regimen should be adjusted for the individual patient. Only then will the optimum elimination of poison be achieved. After rehydrating the patient and correcting any existing acidosis and electrolyte imbalance (particularly hypokalaemia), alkaline diuresis

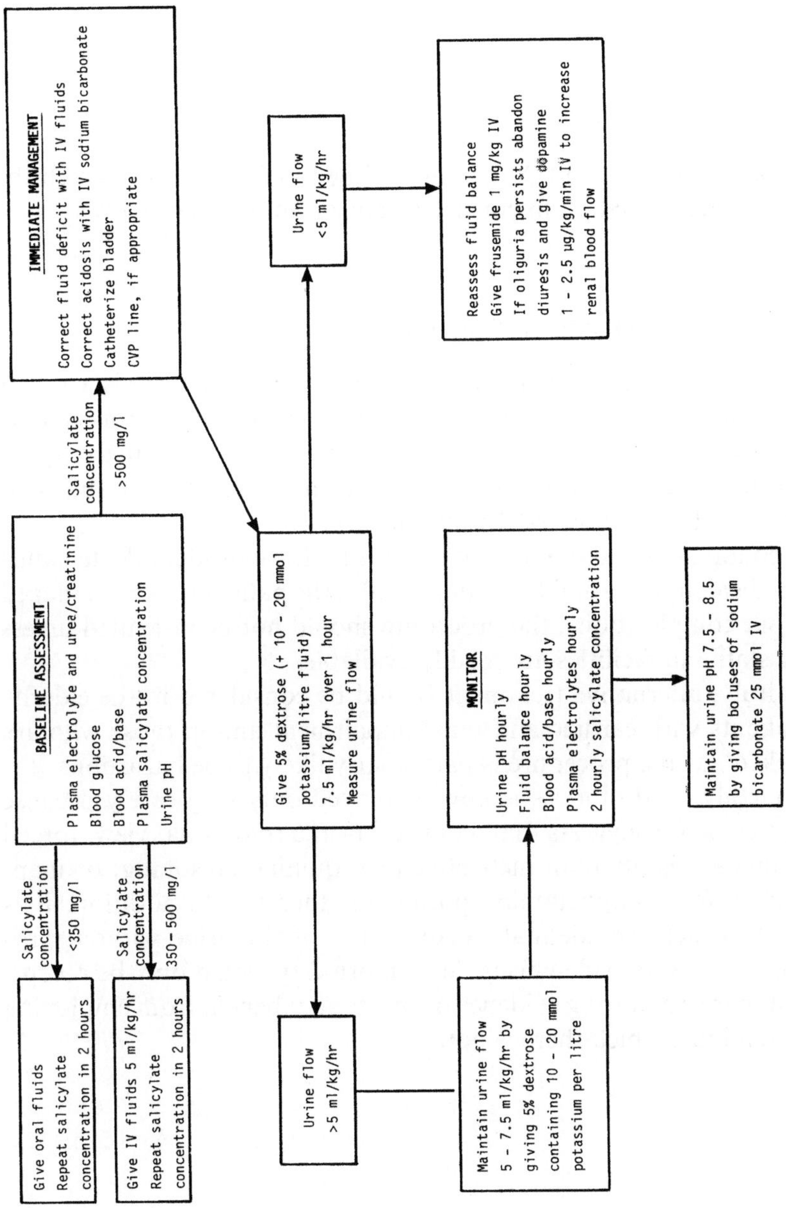

FIGURE 3.2 Procedure for alkaline diuresis in children poisoned with salicylate

should be commenced using the procedures summarized in Figure 3.1 (adults) and Figure 3.2 (children).

Procedure – acid diuresis

The procedure for acid diuresis is outlined in Figure 3.1, though the role for this procedure in clinical practice is minor (see below).

Indications for alkaline and acid diuresis

Contrary to popular belief, the indications for forced diuresis with pH manipulation are few. Firstly, it should be considered only for patients who are clinically poisoned and in whom laboratory analysis has confirmed that an appropriate toxic agent is present in sufficient amount to be the cause of the intoxication.

Secondly, as the use of forced diuresis makes considerable demands on medical, nursing and laboratory staff if the patient is to be managed without complications, the procedure should not be instituted unless these staff and facilities are readily available.

Thirdly, alternative treatment should be considered in the elderly, in patients with cardiac and renal impairment and in those who are 'shocked', as the procedure is particularly likely to be hazardous.

Fourthly, acid diuresis is now employed only very rarely because recent evidence suggests that, contrary to the traditional view, forced acid diuresis is often an ineffective (e.g. quinine poisoning) or inappropriate (e.g. amphetamine poisoning) therapy. In addition, it is difficult to achieve adequate acidification of the urine without producing unpleasant side-effects. Such morbidity would only be acceptable if there was strong evidence of substantial benefit from employing the technique, which there is not.

Forced alkaline diuresis

Phenobarbitone poisoning

Waddell and Butler (1957) demonstrated in dogs that alkalinization of the urine increases the renal clearance of phenobarbitone[15]. Similarly, Bloomer[16] showed that the renal clearance of phenobarbitone rises sharply as the urine pH exceeds 7.5. Prescott has criticized these data[1] and, in studies of his own in poisoned patients, has demonstrated that changes in urinary pH had little effect on tubular reabsorption as shown by the ratio of the urine to plasma concentrations. Moreover, the maximum renal clearance of phenobarbitone achieved by forced alkaline diuresis[17] is of the order of only 17 ml/min, which compares poorly with that found with repeat-dose charcoal therapy.

Salicylate poisoning

The renal clearance of salicylate is dependent on urinary pH. With increasing blood concentrations, the elimination of salicylate by the kidney assumes increasing importance. Morgan and Polak[18] have shown that there is a four-fold increase in renal clearance of salicylate for each rise of one unit in urine pH. Thus, renal salicylate clearance increased from 16 to 64 ml/min as urine pH increased from 6.5 to 7.5. The renal clearance of salicylate also increased with increasing urine flow, an effect that diminished as urine pH rose.

With supportive therapy alone, the plasma elimination half-life of salicylate[14] is approximately 30 h, whereas, with alkaline diuresis, it may be reduced to as little as 6.5 h, even in severely poisoned patients (Figure 3.3).

Phenoxyacetate herbicide poisoning

Alkaline diuresis greatly increases the renal clearance of 2,4-D (2,4-dichlorophenoxyacetic acid) with a concomitant rapid fall in plasma concentration (half-life of 3.7 h compared with 143 h) and corresponding clinical improvement[19]. The effect on mecoprop was similar but less dramatic [19]. These workers showed that, with alkaline diuresis, the renal clearance of 2,4-D rose from 0.14 ml/min to 63 ml/min and that for each increase of 1 pH unit, the renal clearance of 2,4-D rose almost fivefold. In the case of mecoprop, the renal clearance increased twofold for each 1 unit pH rise. More recent evidence[20] confirms the value of alkaline diuresis, not only in the case of 2,4-D and mecoprop, but also in the case of dichlorprop.

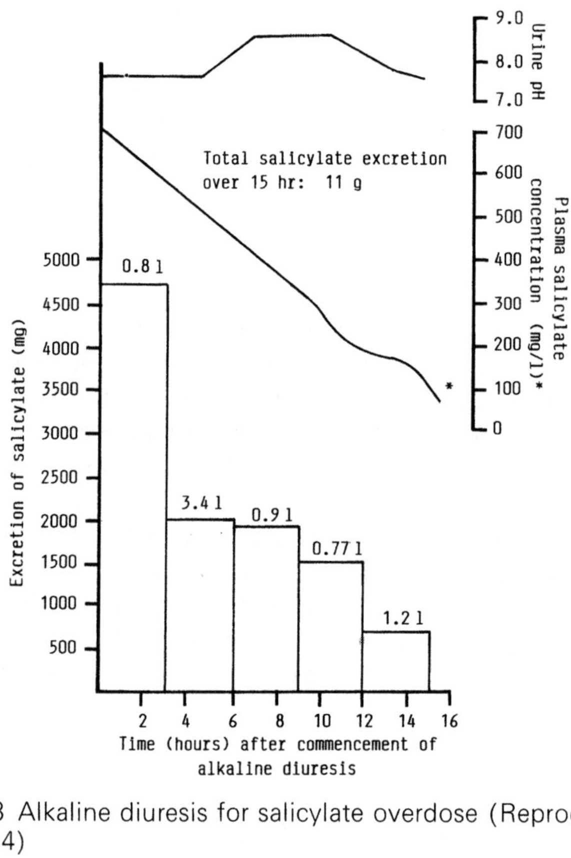

FIGURE 3.3 Alkaline diuresis for salicylate overdose (Reproduced from Reference 44)

Forced acid diuresis

Amphetamine poisoning

Beckett *et al.* demonstrated[21] in volunteers that 57–66% of an administered dose of amphetamine was recovered unchanged in a period of six hours in urines with pH values ranging from 4.8–5.15; less than 5% of the drug was recovered when the urine was alkalinized to a pH of 7.6–8.3. Davis *et al.*[22] have reported a shorter amphetamine plasma half-life (8–10.5 h) with acid (pH 5.5–6.0) urine than with alkaline (pH 7.5–8.0) urine (16–31 h). Anggard *et al.*[23] acidified the urine of three patients and alkalinized the urine of four patients with amphetamine psychosis. The plasma half-life of amphetamine in those with an acid urine was 7–14 h and symptoms cleared rapidly. By contrast, the plasma half-life of the four cases with alkaline urine was 19–34 h and psychosis was prolonged. Gary and Saidi[24] reported data which suggest that acid diuresis increases amphetamine elimination in patients poisoned with amphetamine. Rarely, however, rhabdomyolysis complicates amphetamine intoxication and acid diuresis may increase the risk of the associated renal failure.

Forced acid diuresis is a difficult technique to undertake and, as it may increase morbidity, it should only be considered in those few patients who do not respond to sedation, either with diazepam, chlorpromazine or droperidol.

Fenfluramine poisoning

Urinary acidification increases the renal elimination of fenfluramine[25] but has never been employed widely and there are no published data on which to determine efficacy. Unpublished findings suggest that the amount of drug recovered in the urine is small. Furthermore, sedation with chlorpromazine is invariably sufficient once the risk of early cardiac arrest has passed.

Phencyclidine poisoning

Done[26] showed that acid diuresis increases urinary clearance of phencyclidine from 36 to 271 ml/min, but, surprisingly, there was little effect either on plasma concentration or the time to clinical recovery. Moreover, acid diuresis may potentiate the toxicity of phencyclidine by increasing the risk of renal failure secondary to rhabdomyolysis. Activated charcoal may adsorb phencyclidine and, as this drug is known to diffuse back into the gut after absorption[26], repeat-dose charcoal may be an appropriate alternative.

Quinine poisoning

Recent evidence indicates that quinine elimination cannot be enhanced by the use of acid diuresis[27].

Complications

Fluid overload and hence the precipitation of heart failure, particularly in the elderly, is a common accompaniment of inappropriately managed forced diuresis. Inadequate alkalinization of the urine will result in a poor clinical response and may lead the inexperienced clinician to continue diuresis for several days, with the development of electrolyte and acid–base disturbances, including hypernatraemia, hypokalaemia, hypocalcaemia, hypomagnesaemia and metabolic alkalosis. Although pulmonary oedema in the setting of aspirin poisoning is usually iatrogenic in origin, salicylate itself may induce non-cardiogenic pulmonary oedema. Rarely, cerebral oedema may also occur as a complication of fluid overload.

Conclusion

Alkaline diuresis is appropriate therapy for moderate to severe salicylate poisoning and should also be employed in those who are severely poisoned with phenoxyacetate herbicides. Acid diuresis is unnecessary

unnecessary in the majority of cases of amphetamine, fenfluramine and phencyclidine poisoning and its use may also increase the risk of renal failure. Acid diuresis does not enhance the elimination of quinine.

REPEAT-DOSE CHARCOAL THERAPY

Activated charcoal

Charcoal is prepared from vegetable matter, usually peat, coal, wood, coconut shell and petroleum. Charcoal is 'activated' by heating it at high temperature either in a stream of gas (e.g. steam or carbon dioxide) or with a chemical activating agent, such as phosphoric acid or zinc chloride, or by a combination of both. The process of activation creates a highly developed internal pore structure and thereby increases the surface area from 2–4 m^2/g to an area in excess of 1000 m^2/g; superactivated charcoals (e.g. Super-char (PX21)) have a surface area in excess of 2500 m^2/g.

Mechanism of action

The repeated oral administration of activated charcoal is thought to produce its beneficial effect by:

(1) Adsorbing any unabsorbed toxin still present in the gut. This is particularly relevant in the case of slow-release preparations (e.g. theophylline) or drugs which are slowly absorbed because of decreased gastric motility (e.g. tricyclic antidepressants).

(2) Adsorbing drugs which are secreted in bile, thereby preventing intestinal reabsorption.

(3) Binding any drug which diffuses from the circulation into the gut lumen. After absorption, a drug will re-enter the gut by passive diffusion provided that the concentration there is lower than that in blood. The rate of passive diffusion depends on the concentration gradient and the intestinal surface area, permeability and blood flow. Exceptionally, drugs such as digoxin may, in addition, be actively secreted by the intestinal mucosa, though this

process is unlikely to contribute more than passive diffusion does to the effect of activated charcoal on drug clearance. Under these 'sink' conditions, a concentration gradient is maintained and drug passes continuously into the gut lumen where it is adsorbed.

(4) A purgative action. This may be due either to the addition of sorbitol to charcoal or the use of certain types of charcoal (e.g. Medicoal) which produce diarrhoea rather than severe constipation after the administration of 100–200 g or more (see below).

Factors affecting efficacy

1. Adsorptive capacity of activated charcoal

Although a wide variety of drugs, chemicals and gases can be adsorbed by activated charcoal, several clinically important poisons, e.g. lithium, iron and cyanide are not. Typically, the maximum amounts of substances adsorbed *in vitro* range from 500–1000 mg/g activated charcoal, though superactivated charcoals can adsorb two to three times these amounts. Thus, for a typical adult overdose, substantial quantities (50 g) of activated charcoal must be administered.

2. Amount of charcoal and frequency of administration

For maximum efficiency, charcoal should be given at a rate which firstly, keeps the small intestine filled and, secondly, avoids saturation of the charcoal by exogenous compounds. In a study involving six volunteers, 20 g activated charcoal, given two hourly, produced a significantly greater reduction in the half-life of theophylline than 5 g two hourly[28]. In addition, administering the same total dose of activated charcoal (120 g over 12 hours) in hourly doses rather than less frequently resulted in a further reduction in half-life. The use of inadequate doses of activated charcoal may explain some of the unimpressive results reported, for example in phenobarbitone poisoning (see below).

3. Apparent volume of distribution, tissue binding and half-life of poison

Drugs with a small volume of distribution (< 1 L/kg), low protein and tissue binding and a long half-life, are particularly likely to have their elimination enhanced by repeat doses of activated charcoal. This form of therapy should also be considered when, following overdose, a major route of elimination, such as the kidney, is no longer available due to the onset of organ failure.

4. Difficulties in administration of charcoal
Activated charcoal is unpalatable, due to appearance rather than taste, and administration via a nasogastric tube is therefore almost always necessary in both conscious and unconscious patients. Although activated charcoal increases the elimination of theophylline, salicylate, digoxin and digitoxin (see below), patients poisoned with these drugs may be vomiting (sometimes intractably as in the case of theophylline) and the use of charcoal may therefore be precluded.

Dose and type of charcoal to be employed
It is not known with certainty whether, in poisoned patients, hourly charcoal dosing has therapeutic advantages over 2- or 4-hourly administration, but more frequent administration of smaller doses of charcoal tends to prevent the regurgitation which commonly occurs when large doses are given.

Clinical experience suggests that, after an initial dose of 50–100 g to an adult, charcoal should be administered via a nasogastric tube at a rate of not less than 12.5 g/h. In children, lower doses (10–25 g) of charcoal may be employed because, firstly, smaller overdoses have usually been ingested and, secondly, the gut lumen is narrower.

Superactivated charcoals would appear to offer considerable advantages over other charcoals but they are not yet generally available. An effervescent charcoal preparation (Medicoal), which is available in Europe, has the advantage of a faster transit time than other charcoals such as Carbomix and Norit.

Cathartics: should they be administered at the same time as charcoal?

Cathartics, such a sorbitol, mannitol and sodium and magnesium sulphate, are often given at the same time as activated charcoal in order to:

(1) Increase palatability, e.g. sorbitol sweetens the mixture.
(2) Increase efficacy by decreasing intestinal transit time.
(3) Decrease the risk of severe constipation, which may occur with Carbomix and Norit, but is not usually a major clinical problem unless very large doses (200–500 g) are administered, as may be necessary, for example, in severe phenobarbitone poisoning.

There may be a need to increase palatability if activated charcoal is administered in single doses to prevent poison absorption but it is not realistic to administer charcoal in large and repeated doses without using a nasogastric tube and so palatability is not a prime consideration.

Some animal studies suggest that the co-administration of a cathartic may not only reduce drug adsorption to charcoal but, paradoxically, increase absorption by increasing the volume of intestinal fluid[29]. Furthermore, mannitol and sorbitol delay gastric emptying in man[30], thereby reducing the amount of charcoal available to adsorb the drug in the small bowel.

Recent evidence, however, indicates that, in man, the addition of a cathartic may hasten elimination of a slow-release theophylline preparation from the gut compared with the use of activated charcoal alone[31], though the combined use of sorbitol and charcoal was not without adverse effects. Two of the nine volunteers in this study developed liquid stools, severe abdominal cramps, nausea, sweating and hypotension.

Medicoal alone causes diarrhoea, which may be advantageous in that intestinal transit time is decreased, usually after the administration of some 100–200 g charcoal. It may also be helpful to give Medicoal in combination with either Carbomix or Norit to prevent either profuse diarrhoea or severe constipation.

In summary, the addition of a cathartic may have a therapeutic advantage in emptying the gut of non-absorbed drug, but nursing the patient may be made more difficult. It is possible that the co-administration of a cathartic may reduce the efficacy of activated charcoal by reducing the adsorption of drug to the charcoal. The risk of severe constipation is small unless large doses of a traditional charcoal are administered and, in these circumstances, it is advisable to use either mannitol/sorbitol or to employ Medicoal.

Complications of use

Treatment with repeat-dose activated charcoal is free from serious side-effects, although poor patient acceptability and gastrointestinal complications of use have already been detailed. Pulmonary aspiration of charcoal is rare and does not usually produce clinically significant complications. However, severe airways obstruction has been reported in one infant given charcoal after vomiting was induced by syrup of ipecacuanha[32].

Therapeutic value of repeat-dose activated charcoal

Phenobarbitone poisoning

The value of repeat-dose activated charcoal has been extensively studied in phenobarbitone poisoning. Neuvonen and Elonen[33] gave volunteers activated charcoal at 10, 14, 24, 36 and 48 hours after the oral administration of a therapeutic dose of phenobarbitone and found that the elimination half-life was reduced from a mean of 110 h to 19.8 h. Berg *et al.*[34] subsequently established that the non-renal elimination of *intravenous* phenobarbitone was also significantly increased by repeat-dose charcoal. Goldberg and Berlinger[35] gave repeated oral charcoal to two patients acutely poisoned with phenobarbitone and noted a reduction, not only in the elimination half-life to approximately 24 h, but also in the duration of coma and the need for supportive care.

Pond *et al.*[36] attempted to confirm these findings in a randomized study of 10 comatose patients who required endotracheal intubation and mechanical ventilation. The control and treatment groups both received 50 g activated charcoal on presentation and, in addition, patients in the treatment group were given 17 g activated charcoal together with sorbitol 4 hourly until they had recovered sufficiently to be extubated. Although the mean elimination half-life of phenobarbitone was shortened (Table 3.1), the length of time the patients in each group required mechanical ventilation did not differ significantly and nor did the time spent in hospital. This trial has been criticized as being too small and having unevenly matched groups[37,38]. In addition, the dose of activated charcoal was probably inadequate

TABLE 3.1 Repeat-dose charcoal therapy: phenobarbitone

Reference	*On anticonvulsant therapy* (%)	*Plasma phenobarb. conc.* (mg/L)	*AC total dose* (g)	*AC rate* (g/h)	*Cathartic*	$t_{\frac{1}{2}} \pm SD$ (h)	*Time to recover consciousness* (h)
35	100	141	240	12	Yes	24 approx	22
		107	180	6	Yes		30
36	100	121 ± 31 (*n* = 5)	?	4.25	Yes	36 ± 13	48 ± 8 (to extubation)
39	33	139 ± 76 (*n* = 6)	225–500	15.6–18.75	No	11.7 ± 3.5	16 ± 9

and the co-administration of a cathartic may have reduced the efficacy of activated charcoal.

In another series[39], charcoal in larger doses given without cathartic (Table 3.1), not only greatly enhanced the elimination of phenobarbitone, but also decreased the time to recovery. It should be noted that only one third of the patients in this series were receiving long-term anticonvulsant therapy in contrast to the two previous studies (Table 3.1); enzyme induction is not, therefore, the explanation for the more impressive reduction in half-life. A fourth study[40] employed both alkaline diuresis and repeat-dose activated charcoal in three adolescents and found a mean elimination half-life of 12.3 ± 1.3 h during treatment.

TABLE 3.2 Effect of therapy on phenobarbitone clearance

Treatment	*Penobarbitone clearance* (ml/min)	*Reference*
Untreated	4	142
Forced alkaline diuresis	15	143
Haemodialysis	60	66
Haemoperfusion	77	135
Repeat-dose oral AC	84	39

The value of repeat-dose activated charcoal in phenobarbitone poisoning may be judged by comparing the efficacy of various therapies on drug clearance (Table 3.2); charcoal therapy is the most impressive and the simplest to initiate.

Carbamazepine poisoning

In a randomized cross-over study[33], in 5 volunteers given 400 mg carbamazepine orally, the elimination half-life was reduced from 32 to 17.6 h following repeat-dose charcoal therapy. Boldy *et al.*[41] have shown that charcoal therapy increases carbamazepine clearance in poisoned patients when compared with similarly intoxicated cases[42,43] treated with supportive measures alone (Table 3.3). Oral charcoal therapy is as effective as charcoal haemoperfusion and superior to dialysis (see below) as judged by the total body clearance of carbamazepine.

Salicylate poisoning

The elimination of salicylate is concentration dependent and it is therefore often difficult to compare the results of supportive therapy, repeat-dose charcoal and alkaline diuresis. With supportive therapy alone, the plasma elimination half-life of salicylate may be as long as 30 h[14], whereas, with alkaline diuresis, it may be reduced to 6.5 h even in severely poisoned patients[44].

Hillman and Prescott[45] first reported the value of repeated oral charcoal in enhancing salicylate elimination and their results are compared in Table 3.4 with a series of patients treated in the West Midlands Poisons Unit, Birmingham; two of these latter patients have been reported previously[46].

It should be noted that the patients of Hillman and Prescott all had plasma salicylate concentrations below 500 mg/L at the time that charcoal therapy was commenced, whereas those in the Birmingham series were more severely poisoned. This may explain the longer elimination half-life in the latter group (9.7 ± 3.0 h) compared with the group treated by Hillman and Prescott (3.2 h).

Although repeat-dose charcoal is less metabolically invasive than alkaline diuresis, its use may not be possible in severely vomiting patients even if a nasogastric tube is employed. In severe salicylate poisoning, a well-conducted alkaline diuresis decreases the elimination half-life more rapidly than repeat-dose charcoal therapy but it may be appropriate to employ the latter as an adjunct. Two patients so treated have recently been reported by Mofenson *et al.*[40]. The respective salicylate elimination half-lives were 7.7 and 12.7 h (Table 3.4). In both patients, the plasma concentrations exhibited non-linear disposition, consistent with Michaelis–Menten kinetics, until between 36 and 41h post-ingestion when they changed to first order kinetics.

Theophylline poisoning

Both volunteer (Table 3.5) and clinical studies in poisoned patients (Table 3.6) suggest that repeat-dose charcoal increases clearance and decreases the plasma half-life of theophylline. Theophylline elimination is concentration dependent and this, together with the differing doses of charcoal administered, is thought to explain the variability of half-lives found in practice (Table 3.6). Haemoperfusion and haemodialysis may be more effective than activated charcoal. More-

TABLE 3.3 Repeat-dose charcoal (AC) therapy: carbamazepine (CBZ)

Reference	*Mean maximum CBZ conc.* (mg/L)	*Mean total AC dose* (g)*	*Mean AC rate* (g/h)	$t_{\frac{1}{2}} \pm$ SD (h)	*Body clearance CBZ* (ml/min)
42 (*n*=12)	31.89 ± 5.33 (*n*=10)	Supportive measures only		19.0 ± 6.9†	—
43 (*n*=5)	39.8 ± 22.8	Supportive measures only		18.9 ± 9.8	—
41 (*n*=15)	30.5 ± 12.1	202 ± 58	19.8 ± 11.3	8.6 ± 2.3†	113 ± 44

† $p < 0.001$
* No cathartic

TABLE 3.4 Repeat-dose charcoal (AC) therapy: salicylate

Reference	*n*	*AC rate* (g/h)	$t_{\frac{1}{2}} \pm SD$ (h)
Boldy and Vale (unpublished)	7	>12.5	9.7 ± 3.0
>500 mg/L			
45	5	>12.5	'Mean maximum' 3.2
<500 mg/L			
40	2	15	7.7 ± 1.05
>829 mg/L		(+ $MgSO_4$)	
(+ Alkalinization)			12.7 ± 1.16

over, it is often difficult to employ repeat-dose charcoal therapy because of intractable theophylline-induced vomiting.

Digoxin and digitoxin poisoning

There is evidence from a volunteer study[47] and from studies in poisoned patients[48,49] that repeat doses of activated charcoal increase digoxin elimination. Similarly, the elimination of digitoxin is also increased by these means[50,51]. In practice, vomiting may preclude this therapeutic approach. In addition, in severe cases, the use of digoxin-specific antibody Fab fragments would be more appropriate.

Meprobamate poisoning

Repeat-dose activated charcoal appears to reduce the elimination half-life of meprobamate[52].

Dapsone poisoning

Neuvonen *et al.*[53,54] have demonstrated a reduction in the elimination half-life of dapsone after repeat doses of activated charcoal in both volunteers and three poisoned patients.

Phenylbutazone poisoning

Data from a volunteer study[33] indicate that repeat-dose activated charcoal reduces the plasma half-life of phenylbutazone. No data on poisoned patients have been published.

TABLE 3.5 Theophylline poisoning: repeat-dose activated charcoal (AC): volunteer studies

Reference	*Aminophylline dose IV* (mg/kg)	*AC rate* (g/h)	$t_{\frac{1}{2}} \pm$ SD (h) *Control*	$t_{\frac{1}{2}} \pm$ SD (h) *AC*
144 (*n*=6)	6	23.3	6.4±1.2	3.3±0.4
145 (*n*=7)	8	7.5	10.2±2.1	4.6±1.3
28 (*n*=6)	6	10	9.1±0.7	4.3±0.2
146 (*n*=5)	6	11.7	12.7±4.0	4.0±0.7

TABLE 3.6 Theophylline poisoning: repeat-dose activated charcoal (AC)

Reference	*n*	*Peak plasma concentrations* (mg/L)	*AC rate* (g/h)	$t_{\frac{1}{2}} \pm$SD (h)
146	5	32–59	10	4.9 ± 1.5
147	4	26–50	7.5–15	8.0 ± 3.4
148	10	31–49	15	5.6 ± 2.5
Vale (unpublished)	3	70–288	15–22	4.3 ± 1.3

Tricyclic antidepressant poisoning

A variable effect has been reported on the elimination of tricyclic antidepressants. In volunteer studies, plasma half-lives of amitriptyline and doxepin appear to be reduced unlike that of imipramine[55–57]. It is unlikely, though, that any clinically useful reduction in the elimination half-life of these drugs will be achieved because of their very large volumes of distribution.

Diazepam poisoning

The elimination half-life of diazepam was reduced from 195 to 18 h as a result of charcoal administration in a patient with liver disease treated for delirium tremens with intravenous phenobarbitone and diazepam[58]. Except in such special circumstances, treatment other than supportive measures is not likely to be required for benzodiazepine poisoning. If it is, the use of flumazenil is a simpler, though often more expensive, approach.

Nadolol poisoning

In a volunteer study, the elimination half-life of nadolol was reduced from 17.3 ± 1.7 to 11.8 ± 1.6 h by small doses of activated charcoal given over 9 h[59]. The relevance of this observation to the treatment of poisoned patients is doubtful.

Cyclosporin poisoning

The administration of activated charcoal at a rate of 15 g/h reduced the half-life of cyclosporin from 9 h to 2.5 h in a patient given 5 g by mistake following a transcription error[60].

Conclusion

Repeat-dose activated charcoal has been shown to enhance the non-renal elimination of phenobarbitone, carbamazepine, theophylline, salicylate, dapsone, diazepam, digitoxin, digoxin, meprobamate, phenylbutazone and cyclosporin. As yet, because of the difficulty in conducting large clinical trials, repeat-dose charcoal therapy has not been shown to effect a reduction in either the morbidity or mortality in patients poisoned with these drugs. Further studies are therefore required to establish the role of this interesting new form of treatment and to define the optimum doses of activated charcoal that should be administered.

On the basis of experience to date, activated charcoal should be given at a rate of at least 12.5 g/h via a nasogastric tube after an initial dose of 50–100 g and continued until the patient has recovered or plasma drug concentrations have fallen to safe levels.

Repeat-dose activated charcoal is a simple and relatively inexpensive therapy which appears to be effective for many types of intoxication. In selected patients, it may be preferable to alkaline diuresis, haemoperfusion or haemodialysis.

DIALYSIS

Indications

(1) The drug or toxic substance should diffuse easily through the peritoneum or dialysis membrane.
(2) A significant proportion of the poison should be present in plasma water or capable of rapid equilibration with this compartment.
(3) The toxic effects of the poison should be directly related to the blood concentration.

(4) Dialysis should add significantly to other body mechanisms of elimination.

Peritoneal dialysis

Although widely available, peritoneal dialysis is at least two-to-three times less effective than haemodialysis for the removal of poisons and, since the delivery of toxins to the peritoneum is dependent on blood-flow rate, the efficiency of this technique is reduced in the presence of hypotension. For agents in which metabolism contributes significantly to the total body clearance, dialysate clearance is low and removal by this means is therefore of little importance. Thus, even in the presence of renal failure, peritoneal dialysis has very limited application.

Haemodialysis

Haemodialysis was first used in 1913 for the removal of salicylic acid in experimental poisoning[61] but was not applied clinically until 1950 when it was used for the treatment of salicylate poisoning[62]. It was widely employed during the following two decades and, as a result, there are many reports of its apparent value in the treatment of acute poisoning[63]. Many of these accounts, however, are little more than anecdotal, or even self-adulatory, on the part of the authors. They commonly suffer from a dearth of analytical observations to support the published conclusions. Prescott[1] has examined data purporting to demonstrate the efficacy of haemodialysis and has shown that this method of treatment has often been carried out in patients who have had less than therapeutic plasma concentrations of a drug, or that amounts equivalent to little more than one tablet have been removed.

VALUE OF DIALYSIS

Barbiturate intoxication

The clearance of barbiturate with peritoneal dialysis rarely exceeds 10 ml/min[64,65] which, in the case of phenobarbitone, is unimpressive compared with values achieved by repeat-dose charcoal theapy (Table 3.2). Although phenobarbitone clearance during haemodialysis is greater[66,67], repeat-dose charcoal is again superior (Table 3.2). Short- and medium-acting barbiturates are not amenable to haemodialysis because of their high lipid solubility and protein binding.

Ethchlorvynol poisoning

Mean clearance values of 18.5 ml/min and 64 ml/min were found in one study during peritoneal and haemodialysis, respectively[68]. Haemoperfusion is more efficient.

Glutethimide poisoning

Peritoneal dialysis and haemodialysis are unimpressive and produce clearance values of only 17 ml/min[69] and 34–63 ml/min[70], respectively, though higher values have been reported occasionally[69]. Haemoperfusion is preferred.

Intoxication due to trichloroethanol derivatives

Chloral hydrate is metabolized to trichloroethanol and trichloroacetic acid. There are no data on the efficacy of peritoneal dialysis but clearances of 120–162 ml/min have been achieved during haemodialysis[71,72].

Meprobamate poisoning

Mouton *et al.*[73] have reported that peritoneal dialysis will produce a clearance of only 27 ml/min. Haemodialysis is more impressive and clearances as high as 62 ml/min have been found[74].

Carbamazepine poisoning

Since carbamazepine is extensively metabolized and highly protein bound, peritoneal and haemodialysis are of little value in enhancing its elimination[75,76]; repeat-dose charcoal is as effective or superior[41].

Salicylate poisoning

Peritoneal dialysis has been shown to lower plasma salicylate concentrations. Although less efficient than alkaline diuresis, it can be employed in the presence of renal impairment. Haemodialysis is four times more effective[77].

Poisoning due to alcohols and glycols

Ethanol intoxication

A calculated dialysate clearance of 10–20 ml/min was achieved during peritoneal dialysis in a patient who presented with a blood ethanol concentration of 15 000 mg/L and survived[78]. Haemodialysis is the preferred elimination technique in that it is more efficient than both peritoneal dialysis and charcoal haemoperfusion and it should be considered if the blood ethanol concentration is >500 mg/L and/or if severe metabolic acidosis is present.

Methanol poisoning

During experimental methanol intoxication in dogs, the spontaneous half-life of over 70 h was reduced by a factor of 10 with peritoneal dialysis[79]. Peritoneal dialysis removes three times as much methanol as renal excretion and haemodialysis about 25 times[79]. Keyvan-Larijarni and Tannenberg[80] reported the value of peritoneal dialysis in three patients with admission blood methanol concentrations ranging from 960–1980 mg/L. After eight hours, a 13% reduction in methanol concentration was achieved compared with a 66% reduction by haemodialysis in other patients. One death and one case of permanent blindness occurred in those treated by peritoneal dialysis whereas all patients treated by haemodialysis survived.

Due to its low molecular weight (32 Da), lack of protein-binding and low volume of distribution (0.7 L/kg), methanol is easily removed by haemodialysis[81]. The clearance values lie between 150–200 ml/min depending on the blood flow and surface area of the dialyser. In addition, haemodialysis may also remove formate[82,83]; clearance values range from 140–150 ml/min.

Ethylene glycol poisoning

Vale *et al.*[84] showed that peritoneal dialysis removes ethylene glycol, albeit at a slower rate than haemodialysis. Since ethylene glycol has a low molecular weight (62 Da), low protein binding and a volume of distribution of 0.7–0.8 L/kg, this glycol ought to be dialysable though it is less so than methanol[85–87]. Recently, the dialysance of glycolate (140 ml/min), a metabolite of ethylene glycol, has also been demonstrated in one patient[88].

Isopropanol poisoning

Isopropanol has a small molecular weight, low volume of distribution and low plasma protein binding and dialysis is therefore likely to be successful. Peritoneal dialysis is considerably less effective than haemodialysis, both in removing isopropanol and in shortening the duration of coma in those intoxicated[89–93].

Lithium intoxication

Lithium can be removed by peritoneal dialysis[5,94], though this technique is less efficient than haemodialysis. Clearances of 13–15 ml/min have been achieved with peritoneal dialysis[95] compared with haemodialysis clearance values of 60–132 ml/min[5,6,95–98]. However, after haemodialysis, there is often a rebound increase in serum lithium concentration due to the slow diffusion of lithium across cell membranes. Haemodialysis is the treatment of choice in severe lithium intoxication though there has been debate recently on when it should be employed and for what period[99,100]. Following an acute overdose of lithium, haemodialysis may prevent lithium diffusion into the brain and the onset of severe toxicity. In contrast, those patients who develop intoxication during chronic therapy may require long periods of dialysis to produce clinical improvement.

Theophylline poisoning

Peritoneal dialysis produces a theophylline clearance of the same order as the endogenous clearance rate: in children aged 18 months and 34 months old, it was 1.3 ml/min and 5.1 ml/min, respectively[101,102]. In addition, Brown *et al.*[103] found that theophylline clearance in adults during dialysis was less than 12 ml/min; only 4 mg was removed over a 48 h period. Lee *et al.*[104] reported similar values (9.5 ml/min). Thus, peritoneal dialysis is much less effective than haemodialysis which can achieve clearances of 112 ml/min[105] in adults if blood flow is maintained. When it is not, clearances between 33 and 88 ml/min are obtained[106,107]. Haemodialysis can, therefore, be expected to double the total body clearance of theophylline but is less effective than haemoperfusion (see below).

Conclusion

Haemodialysis is an efficient technique for the removal of salicylate, ethanol, methanol, ethylene glycol, isopropanol and lithium.

HAEMOPERFUSION

Development

Haemoperfusion involves the passage of blood through devices containing adsorbent particles, usually activated charcoal or uncharged resins, such as Amberlite XAD-4, to which drugs are adsorbed by surface forces.

In 1965, Yatzidis and his colleagues in Greece[108] perfused the blood of two patients poisoned by barbiturates through an uncoated charcoal system. Good drug removal was achieved but a number of complications ensued, including charcoal embolism, marked thrombocytopenia, fibrinogen loss and pyrogen reactions. Attempts were subsequently made to eliminate these adverse effects by coating the carbon with a biocompatible polymer. Chang *et al.*[109], for example, utilized cellulose nitrate and albumin as a coating and perfused three patients. Vale *et al.*[110,111] successfully perfused 20 patients using a device containing 300 g polyhydroxyethylmethacrylate-coated carbon and this system was subsequently made available commercially by Smith and Nephew as Haemacol. Later, a device containing cellulose acetate-coated carbon was marketed (Absorba 300C, Gambro) and an even more recent development has been the introduction of systems using petroleum-based activated carbon beads which are extremely hard and very resistant to mechanical abrasion[112].

In the early 1960s, several workers investigated the use of anion-exchange resins in an attempt to reduce or eliminate the haematological and other adverse effects which were common with uncoated charcoal devices. Complications persisted, however, but Rosenbaum *et al.*[113] introduced a resin system using Amberlite XAD-4 and, subsequently, a cartridge containing 650 g XAD-4 was released for clinical use (Extracorporeal).

Indications

The indications for haemoperfusion are based on general and clinical considerations.

Clinical considerations

Although the overall mortality of poisoned patients is less than 1%, that of patients who present in grade 4 coma following an overdose of a barbiturate or non-barbiturate hypnotic, ranges from 5–40%. The mortality following severe theophylline poisoning may also be high despite excellent supportive care. Based on these considerations, the following criteria for haemoperfusion were agreed by a multicentre group in Great Britain in 1974. A patient should meet three of the following criteria:

(1) Be severely poisoned, as shown for example by grade 4 coma, hypotension, hypothermia and hypoventilation following the ingestion of hypnotic drugs.
(2) Suffer progressive clinical deterioration despite the best supportive management.
(3) Show no evidence of improvement despite full resuscitative measures.
(4) Suffer prolonged coma and complications such as pneumonia, shocked lung, or underlying chronic respiratory disease.
(5) Have high plasma concentrations of the toxic agent.

General considerations

The main considerations are that:

(1) The toxic substance should be readily adsorbed on to charcoal or resin.
(2) A significant proportion of the poison should be present in plasma water or capable of rapid equilibration with it.
(3) The toxic effects of the poison should be directly related to the blood concentration.
(4) Haemoperfusion should add significantly to other body mechanisms of elimination.

Contraindications

Haemoperfusion is contraindicated if:

(1) The poison has a very large volume of distribution.
(2) An antidote or protective agent is available, as it is, for example, for opiates, paracetamol, β-adrenoceptor-blocking drugs, digoxin, cyanide, organophosphorus insecticides.
(3) The poison acts very rapidly, e.g. cyanide.
(4) The drug ingested is relatively non-toxic, e.g. benzodiazepines.
(5) The effects of the toxin are irreversible, e.g. in the late phase of poisoning due to organophosphorus insecticides.
(6) Haemodialysis is more effective as it is in removing salicylate, ethylene glycol, ethanol, methanol, isopropanol and lithium.

Efficacy

The major rate-limiting factors in removal of toxins by haemoperfusion are the affinity of the adsorbent for the toxin, the rate of blood flow through the circuit, the volume of distribution of the toxin and the rate of equilibration of toxin from tissues to blood. Haemoperfusion is more efficient than haemodialysis in removing barbiturates and non-barbiturate hypnotics (see below), though there are differences between the performance of haemoperfusion systems using activated charcoal and XAD-4 resin. Activated charcoal adsorbs both polar and non-polar drugs, but XAD-4 resin removes most non-polar drugs more efficiently than charcoal.

Haemoperfusion over 4–6 h significantly reduces the body burden of compounds with a low volume of distribution (<1 L/kg). For compounds with intermediate values (2–6 L/kg), longer periods of haemoperfusion are necessary. Haemoperfusion cannot reduce significantly the body burden of those poisons which have very large volumes of distribution. Furthermore, although toxin clearance during haemoperfusion is a general guide to the efficacy of the technique, it may be misleading if only a small proportion of the body load of poison is removed. For example, death will still ensue if a substantial amount of paraquat is ingested, even though haemoperfusion is performed and the clearances achieved are impressive; the amount of paraquat removed is a fraction of the dose ingested.

Haemoperfusion has been used to treat patients poisoned with β-adrenoceptor-blocking drugs, camphor, digoxin, mercury, opiates, organophosphorus compounds, paraquat, quinine and diazepam, though its value in these cases is very questionable. There is, however, good evidence that haemoperfusion effectively removes barbiturates, carbamazepine, disopyramide, ethchlorvynol, glutethimide, meprobamate, theophylline and trichloroethanol derivatives. The role of haemoperfusion in these cases will be considered below.

Efficacy may be judged in three ways:

(1) Clearance during haemoperfusion may be compared with endogenous clearance and that achieved by other elimination techniques.
(2) The amount of toxin removed during haemoperfusion. Does this represent a substantial proportion of the total body load?
(3) A reduction in morbidity and mortality.

There is now considerable clinical experience of haemoperfusion[109–123], and its value has been reviewed[63,124,125]. Charcoal haemoperfusion has been employed more frequently than resin haemoperfusion, not least because it is often difficult to achieve prolonged blood flow satisfactorily through a resin system.

Unfortunately, comparison between published studies is difficult as the authors often do not include detailed kinetic data or give only the maximum clearance value achieved which may not be typical. The evaluation of haemoperfusion given below is based on published data and extensive personal experience of the technique.

Barbiturate poisoning

There is good evidence that charcoal and resin haemoperfusion produce more impressive drug clearances than endogenous elimination alone, alkaline diuresis, or dialysis (Table 3.7). However, recent work[39] has demonstrated that repeat-dose activated charcoal is as efficient as charcoal haemoperfusion in the case of phenobarbitone intoxication.

TABLE 3.7 Mean clearance (ml/min) achieved by forced diuresis (FD), peritoneal dialysis (PD), haemodialysis (HD) and haemoperfusion(HP)

Drug	*FD**	*PD**	*HD**	*HP***
Amylobarbitone	5	10	30	75
Butobarbitone	5	10	30	75
Phenobarbitone	20	10	60	77
Meprobamate	—	27	62	125
Glutethimide	—	17	50	125
Ethchlorvynol	20	18.5	64	184
Trichloroethanol	—	—	120–162	186–221

* Data obtained from literature
**From references 110 and 111 and unpublished data

Glutethimide poisoning

Haemoperfusion results in a more impressive drug clearance than haemodialysis (Table 3.7). A significant rebound in plasma concentration occurs in some patients and repeated haemoperfusion may be necessary.

Ethchlorvynol poisoning

Resin haemoperfusion effectively removes ethchlorvynol and is superior to haemodialysis[126] (Table 3.7).

Meprobamate poisoning

Clearance values of 80–300 ml/min have been achieved using charcoal and resin haemoperfusion with very high blood flow rates[114]. These values are superior to those achieved by peritoneal and haemodialysis (Table 3.7).

Poisoning due to trichloroethanol derivatives

Mean haemoperfusion clearances of 198 ± 20 ml/min were achieved by De Groot[114]. Haemoperfusion is therefore more effective than haemodialysis in removing trichloroethanol and its derivatives.

Carbamazepine poisoning

Charcoal haemoperfusion has been shown to produce clearance values of 80–129 ml/min[127–129] and elimination half-lives during perfusion of 8.6–10.7 h[128], though these values are similar to those achieved by repeat-dose activated charcoal therapy[41].

Theophylline poisoning

Heath and Knudsen[130] have recently reviewed the value of haemoperfusion in theophylline poisoning. They conclude that 'of the invasive techniques available, charcoal haemoperfusion is the most effective, increasing clearance four-fold'. Haemoperfusion should be *considered* if plasma concentrations are greater than 100 mg/L following an acute overdose or greater than 60 mg/L in a patient receiving theophylline chronically. However, the use of supportive measures (including the correction of electrolyte and metabolic abnormalities) and repeat-dose oral activated charcoal usually obviates the need for haemoperfusion.

Disopyramide poisoning

There is evidence that Amberlite XAD-4 resin (but not charcoal) haemoperfusion together with inotropic support may increase elimination sufficiently to prevent a fatal outcome in cases of severe poisoning[131], though inotropic support alone may be sufficient, even in very severely poisoned patients.

Phenylbutazone poisoning

In an *in vivo* study, Okonek[132] found XAD-4 resin haemoperfusion to be unimpressive in removing phenylbutazone. However, it has been employed clinically[133,134] and success for its use claimed. Clinical experience is too limited to know whether haemoperfusion is more effective than repeat-dose activated charcoal.

Does haemoperfusion reduce morbidity and mortality?

Of a series of 28 patients suffering from barbiturate and non-barbiturate hypnotic drug poisoning who were haemoperfused between 1973 and 1977, all but six recovered[135]. Four of those who died suffered hypoxic brain damage as a result of a cardiorespiratory arrest prior to haemoperfusion; another developed atrial fibrillation after the discontinuation of haemoperfusion and subsequently developed hemiplegia and the sixth patient, who was a diabetic, recovered completely but subsequently developed bronchopneumonia and died 15 days later. Despite these patients being highly selected and thus very severely poisoned, the mortality was only 21% compared with 34% in an unselected series of cases given intensive supportive therapy alone[136]. In addition, the duration of coma was greatly shortened[135].

Complications of haemoperfusion

The complications of haemoperfusion are summarized in Table 3.8.

There is a fall of approximately 30% in the platelet count and a fall of up to 10% in the leukocyte count, both of which are maximal within the first hour. Thereafter, they return to normal values. These reductions are similar to those seen during other extracorporeal procedures, such as haemodialysis and cardiac bypass surgery. It is known that the degree of thrombocytopenia depends on the rate of blood flow, the presence or absence, type and thickness of the coating in the perfusion system and the type of adsorbent material used in the haemoperfusion column. Two mechanisms have been postulated to explain the thrombocytopenia:

TABLE 3.8 Potential complications of haemoperfusion

Haemorrhage because of heparinization
Patient may disconnect shunt lines
Air embolism
Infection
Loss of peripheral artery
Thrombocytopenia, leukopenia
Loss of clotting factors
$Ca^{2+}\downarrow$ Glucose$\downarrow$ Urea$\downarrow$ Creatinine$\downarrow$ Urate$\downarrow$

(1) The loss and possible destruction of platelets in the extracorporeal circuit. When blood comes into contact with the extracorporeal system, ADP and serotonin are released and result in platelet aggregation. The more adhesive members of the platelet population ('sticky platelets') are removed in the first few minutes after perfusion is commenced and no further fall in the count occurs if the lines and perfusion column are changed. Moreover, it is known that platelet adhesiveness falls during extracorporeal procedures[137].

(2) The reversible sequestration of platelets in the liver and possibly in the spleen[138].

The fall in platelet count may be reduced by the administration of sulphinpyrazone[77] and prostacyclin[139,140] but not by aspirin[77].

Generally, no biochemical changes of clinical significance occur, though there is often a fall in the plasma glucose level on commencing haemoperfusion and this is most noticeable with the DHD-1 column (Kuraray). Transient hypocalcaemia has also been reported with this same column, and intravenous calcium was required throughout the procedure in one patient[112]. Small falls in plasma urate, urea, creatinine, bilirubin, phosphate and cholesterol levels have also been observed with other haemoperfusion systems.

Conclusion

Haemoperfusion is a safe procedure to institute and maintain and may be continued for long periods without serious complications ensuing provided that the clinician concerned is experienced in its use. It is particularly valuable in severely poisoned patients who have ingested a barbiturate or non-barbiturate hypnotic (excluding phenobarbitone), theophylline, disopyramide or phenylbutazone, and who have failed to improve despite the use of supportive measures. Haemoperfusion may reduce the morbidity and mortality in patients severely poisoned with barbiturates and non-barbiturate hypnotics and this may well be true for theophylline as well. Haemoperfusion may also have a diagnostic role in the management of patients in prolonged coma who have suffered a cardiorespiratory arrest and who have high plasma drug concentrations of one of the agents mentioned above.

REFERENCES

1. Prescott, L.F. (1974). Limitations of haemodialysis and forced diuresis. In *The Poisoned Patient: The Role of the Laboratory,* Ciba Foundation Symposium No. 26, pp. 269–282. (Amsterdam: North Holland/Excerpta Medica)
2. Bochner, F., Hooper, W.D., Sutherland, J.M., Eadie, M.J. and Tyner, J. (1973). The renal handling of diphenylhydration and 5-(p-hydroxyphenol)-5-phenylhydration. *Clin. Pharm. Ther.* **14,** 791–796
3. Richens, A. (1979). Clinical pharmacokinetics of phenytoin. *Clin. Pharmacokinet.,* **4,** 153–169
4. Thomsen, K. (1973). The effect of sodium chloride on kidney function in rats with lithium intoxication. *Acta Pharmacol. Toxicol.,* **33,** 92–102
5. Hansen, H.E. and Amdisen, A. (1978). Lithium intoxication. *Q. J. Med.,* **47,** 123–144
6. Jacobsen, D., Aarsen, G., Frederichsen, P. and Eisenga, B. (1987). Lithium intoxication: pharmacokinetics during and after terminated haemodialysis in acute intoxications. *Clin. Toxicol.,* **25,** 81–94
7. Dyson, E.H., Simpson, D., Prescott, L.F. and Proudfoot, A.T. (1987). Self-poisoning and therapeutic intoxication with lithium. *Human Toxicol.,* **6,** 325–329
8. Macdonald, T.M., Cotton, M. and Prescott, L.F. (1988). Low dose dopamine in lithium poisoning. *Br. J. Clin. Pharmacol.,* **26,** 195–197
9. Berg, K.J. (1977). Acute acetylsalicylic acid poisoning: Treatment with forced alkaline diuresis and diuretics. *Eur. J. Clin. Pharm.,* **12,** 111–116
10. Cumming, G., Dukes, D.C. and Widdowson, G. (1964). Alkaline diuresis in treatment of aspirin poisoning. *Br. Med. J.,* **2,** 1033–1036
11. Dukes, D.C., Blainey, J.D., Cumming, G. and Widdowson, G. (1963). The treatment of severe aspirin poisoning. *Lancet,* **1,** 329–331
12. Lawson, A.A.H., Proudfoot, A.T., Brown, S.S., Macdonald, H., Fraser, A.G., Cameron, J.C. and Matthew, H. (1969). Forced diuresis in the treatment of acute salicylate poisoning in adults. *Q. J. Med.,* **38,** 31–48

13. Meredith, T. J. and Vale, J. A. (1981). Salicylate poisoning. In Vale, J. A. and Meredith, T. J. (eds.) *Poisoning: Diagnosis and Treatment,* pp. 97–103. (London: Update Books)
14. Prescott, L. F., Balali-Mood, M., Critchley, J. A. J. H., Johnstone, A. F. and Proudfoot, A. T. Diuresis or urinary alkalinisation for salicylate poisoning. *Br. Med. J.,* **285,** 1383–1386
15. Waddell, W. J. and Butler, T. C. (1957). The distribution and excretion of phenobarbital. *J. Clin. Invest.,* **36,** 1217–1226
16. Bloomer, H. A. (1966). A critical evaluation of diuresis in the treatment of barbiturate intoxication. *J. Lab. Clin. Med.,* **67,** 898–905
17. Hadden, J., Johnson, K., Smith, S., Price, L. and Giardina, E. (1969). Acute barbiturate intoxication: Concepts of management. *J. Am. Med. Soc.,* **209,** 893–900
18. Morgan, A. G. and Polak, A. (1971). The excretion of salicylate in salicylate poisoning. *Clin. Sci.,* **41,** 475–484
19. Prescott, L. F., Park, J. and Darrien, I. (1979). Treatment of severe 2,4-D and mecoprop intoxication with alkaline diuresis. *Br. J. Clin. Pharm.,* **7,** 111–116
20. Onyon, L. J., Liddle, A. and Flanagan, R. J. (1986). Acute toxicity of chlorinated phenoxy herbicides in man. *Hum. Toxicol.,* **5,** 127–128
21. Beckett, A. H., Rowland, M. and Turner, P. (1965). Influence of urinary pH on excretion of amphetamine. *Lancet,* **1,** 303
22. Davis, J. M., Kopin, I. J., Lemberger, L. and Axelrod, J. (1971). Effects of urinary pH on amphetamine excretion. *Ann. N.Y. Acad. Sci.,***179,** 493–501
23. Anggard, E., Johnson, L.-E., Hogmark, A.-L. and Gunne, L.-M. (1973). Amphetamine metabolism in amphetamine psychosis. *Clin. Pharm. Ther.,* **14,** 870–879
24. Gary, N. E. and Saidi, P. (1978). Methamphetamine intoxication: A speedy new treatment. *Am. J. Med.,* **64,** 537–540
25. Beckett, A. H. and Brookes, L. G. (1967). The absorption and urinary excretion in man of fenfluramine and its main metabolite. *J. Pharm. Pharmacol.,* **19** (Suppl.), 41S–45S
26. Done, A. K. (1980). Ion trapping in the pathogenesis and treatment of poisoning. *Vet. Hum. Toxicol.,* **22** (Suppl 2), 2–9
27. Bateman, D. N., Blain, P. G., Woodhouse, K. W., Rawlins, M. D., Dyson, H., Heyworth, R., Prescott, L. F. and Proudfoot, A. T. (1985). Pharmacokinetics and clinical toxicity of quinine overdosage: Lack of efficacy of techniques intended to enhance elimination. *Q. J. Med.,* **54,** 125–131
28. Park, G. D., Radomski, L., Goldberg, M. J., Spector, R., Johnson, G. F. and Quee, C. K. (1983). Effects of size and frequency of oral doses of charcoal on theophylline clearance. *Clin. Pharm. Ther.,* **34,** 663–666
29. Van de Graaff, W. B., Leigh Thompson, W., Sunshine, I., Fretthold, D., Leickly, F. and Dayton, H. (1982). Adsorbent and cathartic inhibition of enteral drug absorption. *J. Pharmacol. Exp. Ther.,* **221,** 656–663
30. Hunt, J. N. and Stubbs, D. F. (1975). The volume and energy content of meals as determinants of gastric emptying. *J. Physiol.* (*London*), **245,** 209–225
31. Goldberg, M. J., Spector, R., Park, G. D., Johnson, G. F. and Roberts, P. (1987). The effect of sorbitol and activated charcoal on serum theophylline concentrations after slow-release theophylline. *Clin. Pharm. Ther.,* **41,** 108–111
32. Pollock, M. M., Dunbar, B. S., Holbrook, P. R. and Fields, A. I. (1981). Aspir-

ation of activated charcoal and gastric contents. *Ann. Emerg. Med.*, **10**, 528–529

33. Neuvonen, P. J. and Elonen, E. (1980). Effect of activated charcoal on absorption and elimination of phenobarbitone, carbamazepine and phenylbutazone in man. *Eur. J. Clin. Pharmacol.*, **17**, 51–57
34. Berg, M. J., Berlinger, W. G., Goldberg, M. J., Spector, R. and Johnson, G. F. (1982). Acceleration of the body clearance of phenobarbital by oral activated charcoal. *N. Engl. J. Med.*, **307**, 642–644
35. Goldberg, M. J. and Berlinger, W. G. (1982). Treatment of phenobarbital overdose with activated charcoal. *J. Am. Med. Assoc.* **247**, 2400–2401
36. Pond, S. M., Olson, K. R., Osterloh, J. D. and Tong, T. G. (1984). Randomized study of the treatment of phenobarbital overdose with repeated doses of activated charcoal. *J. Am. Med. Assoc.*, **251**, 3104–3108
37. Goldberg, M. J., Berlinger, W. G. and Park, G. D. (1985). Activated charcoal in phenobarbital overdose. *J. Am. Med. Assoc.* **253**, 1120–1121
38. Pond, S. M., Osterloh, J. D., Olson, K. R. and Tong, T. G. (1985). Activated charcoal in phenobarbital overdose. *J. Am. Med. Assoc.*, **253**, 1121
39. Boldy, D. A. R., Vale, J. A. and Prescott, L. F. (1986). Treatment of phenobarbitone poisoning with repeated oral administration of activated charcoal. *Q. J. Med.*, **61**, 997–1002
40. Mofenson, H. C., Caraccio, T. R., Greensher, J., D'Agostino, R. and Rossi, A. (1985). Gastrointestinal dialysis with activated charcoal and cathartic in the treatment of adolescent intoxications. *Clin. Pediatr.*, **24**, 678–684
41. Boldy, D. A. R., Heath, A., Ruddock, S., Vale, J. A. and Prescott, L. F. (1987). Repeated oral activated charcoal in the treatment of carbamazepine poisoning. *Lancet*, **1**, 1027
42. Hundt, H. K. L., Aucamp, A. K. and Muller, F. O. (1983). Pharmacokinetic aspects of carbamazepine and its two major metabolites in plasma during overdosage. *Hum. Toxicol.*, **2**, 607–614
43. Vree, T. B., Janssen, T. J., Hekster, Y. A., Termond, E. F. S., van de Dries, A. C. P. and Wijnands, W. J. A. (1986). Clinical pharmocokinetics of carbamazepine and its epoxy and hydroxy metabolites in humans after an overdose. *Ther. Drug Monitoring*, **8**, 297–304
44. Vale, J. A. and Meredith, T. J. (1981). Forced diuresis, dialysis and haemoperfusion. In Vale, J. A. and Meredith, T. J. (eds.) *Poisoning: Diagnosis and Treatment*. (London: Update Books)
45. Hillman, R. J. and Prescott, L. F. (1985). Treatment of salicylate poisoning with repeated oral charcoal. *Br. Med. J.*, **291**, 1472
46. Boldy, D. and Vale, J. A. (1986). Treatment of salicylate poisoning with repeated oral charcoal. *Br. Med. J.*, **292**, 136
47. Lalonde, R. L., Deshpande, R., Hamilton, P. P., McLean, W. M. and Greenway, D. C. (1985). Acceleration of digoxin clearance by activated charcoal. *Clin. Pharm. Ther.*, **37**, 367–371
48. Boldy, D. A. R., Smart, V. and Vale, J. A. (1985). Multiple doses of charcoal in digoxin poisoning. *Lancet*, **2**, 1076–1077
49. Lake, K. D., Brown, D. C. and Peterson, C. D. (1984). Digoxin toxicity: Enhanced systemic elimination during oral activated charcoal therapy. *Pharmacotherapy*, **4**, 161–163
50. Moulin, M. A., Potier, J. C., Grollier, G. and Camsonne, R. (1982). Intoxication

a la digitoxine: elimination acceleree par administration du charbon actif. *Nouv. Presse Med.*, **11,** 1079–1080

51. Pond, S., Jacobs, M., Marks, J., Garner, J., Goldschlager, N. and Hansen, D. (1981). Treatment of digitoxin overdose with oral activated charcoal. *Lancet,* **2,** 1177–1178
52. Linden, C. H. and Rumack, B. H. (1984). Enhanced elimination of meprobamate by multiple doses of activated charcoal. *Vet. Hum. Toxicol.,* **26** (Suppl. 2), 47
53. Neuvonen, P. J., Elonen, E. and Mattila, M. J. (1980). Oral activated charcoal and dapsone elimination. *Clin. Pharm. Ther.,* **27,** 823–827
54. Neuvonen, P. J., Elonen, E. and Haapanen, E. J. (1983). Acute dapsone intoxication: clinical findings and effect of oral charcoal and haemodialysis on dapsone elimination. *Acta Med. Scand.,* **214,** 215–220
55. Goldberg, M. J., Park, G. D., Spector, R., Fischer, L. J. and Feldman, R. D. (1985). Lack of effect of oral activated charcoal on imipramine clearance. *Clin. Pharmacol. Ther.,* **38,** 350–353
56. Scheinin, M., Virtanen, R. and Iisalo, E. (1985). Effect of single and repeated doses of activated charcoal on the pharmacokinetics of doxepin. *Int. J. Clin. Pharm. Ther. Toxicol,* **23,** 38–42
57. Swartz, C. M. and Sherman, A. (1984). The treatment of tricyclic antidepressant overdose with repeated charcoal. *J. Clin. Psychopharmacol.,* **4,** 336–340
58. Traeger, S. M. and Haug, M. T. (1986). Reduction of diazepam serum half-life and reversal of coma by activated charcoal in a patient with severe liver disease. *Clin. Toxicol.,* **24,** 329–337
59. Du Souich, P., Caille, G. and Larochelle, P. (1983). Enhancement of nadolol elimination by activated charcoal and antibiotics. *Clin. Pharm. Ther.,* **33,** 585–590
60. Honcharik, N. and Anthone, S. (1985). Activated charcoal in acute cyclosporin overdose. *Lancet,* **1,** 1051
61. Abel, J. J., Rowntree, L. G. and Turner, B. B. (1914). On the removal of diffusible substances from the circulating blood of living animals by dialysis. *J. Pharm. Exp. Ther.,* **5,** 275–316
62. Doolan, P. P., Walsh, W. P., Kyle, L. H. and Wishinsky, H. (1951). Acetylsalicylic acid intoxication: A proposed method of treatment. *J. Am. Med. Assoc.* **146,** 105–106
63. Winchester, J. F., Gelfand, M. C., Knepshield, J. H. and Schreiner, G. E. (1977). Dialysis and hemoperfusion of poisons and drug-update. *Trans. Am. Soc. Artif. Intern. Organs,* **23,** 762–842
64. Berman, L. B. and Vogelsang, P. (1964). Removal rates for barbiturates using two types of peritoneal dialysis. *N. Engl. J. Med.* **270,** 77–80
65. Kennedy, A. C., Briggs, J. D., Young, N., Lindsay, R. M., Luke, R. G. and Campbell, D. (1969). Successful treatment of three cases of very severe barbiturate poisoning. *Lancet,* **1,** 995–998
66. Berman, L. B., Jeghers, H. J., Schreiner, G. E. and Pallotta, A. J. (1956). Hemodialysis, an effective therapy for acute barbiturate poisoning. *J. Am. Med. Assoc.,* **161,** 820–827
67. Takki, S., Gambertoglio, J. G., Honda, D. H. and Tozer, T. N. (1978). Pharmacokinetic evaluation of hemodialysis in acute drug overdose. *J. Pharmacokinetic. Biopharm.,* **6,** 427–442
68. Teehan, B. P., Maher, J. F., Carey, J. J. H., Flynn, P. D. and Schreiner, G. E.

(1970). Acute ethchlorvynol (Placidyl) intoxication. *Ann. Intern. Med.*, **72,** 875–882

69. De Myttenaere, M., Schoenfeld, L. and Maher, J. F. (1968). Treatment of glutethimide poisoning. A comparison of forced diuresis and dialysis. *J. Am. Med. Assoc.*, **203,** 165–167
70. Stein, G., Kangas, L., Traeger, A., Sperschneider, H., Funfstuck, R. and Preissler, G. (1977). In-vitro- und in-vivo- Dialysance-Untersuchungen von Psychopharmaka, Hypnotika und Lithium. *Dtsch Gesundh-Wesen,* **32,** 1952–1955
71. Stalker, N. E., Gambertoglio, J. G., Fukumitsu, C. J., Naughton, J. L. and Benet, L. Z. (1978). Acute massive chloral hydrate intoxication treated with hemodialysis: a clinical pharmacokinetic analysis. *J. Clin. Pharmacol.*, **18,** 136–142
72. Vaziri, N. D., Kumar, K. P., Mirahmadi, K. and Rosen, S. M. (1977). Hemodialysis in treatment of acute chloral hydrate poisoning. *South. Med. J.*, **70,** 377–378
73. Mouton, D. E., Cohen, R. J. and Barrett, O'N. (1976). Meprobamate poisoning: successful treatment with peritoneal dialysis. *Am. J. Med. Sci.*, **253,** 706–709
74. Lobo, P. I., Spyker, D., Surratt, P. and Westervelt, F. B. (1977). Use of hemodialysis in meprobamate overdosage. *Clin. Nephrol.*, **7,** 73–75
75. Lee, C.-S.C., Wang, L. H., Marbury, T. C., Bruni, J. and Perchalski, R. J. (1980). Hemodialysis clearance and total body elimination of carbamazepine during chronic hemodialysis. *Clin. Toxicol.*, **17,** 429–438
76. Gruska, H., Peyer, K.-H., Kubicki, S. and Schneider, H. (1971). Klinik toxicologie und Therapie einer Schweren Carbamazepin-vergiftung. *Arch. Toxicol.*, **27,** 193–203
77. Winchester, J. F., Forbes, C. D., Courtney, J. M., Reavey, M. and Prentice, C. R. M. (1977). Effect of sulphinpyrazone and aspirin on platelet adhesion to activated charcoal and dialysis membranes in vitro. *Thromb. Res.*, **11,** 443
78. O'Neill, S., Tipton, K. F., Prichard, J. S. and Quinlan, A. (1984). Survival after high blood alcohol levels: Association with first order elimination kinetics. *Arch. Intern. Med.*, **144,** 641–642
79. Schreiner, G. E. (1970). Dialysis of poisons and drugs – annual review. *Trans. Am. Soc. Artif. Intern. Org.*, **16,** 544–568
80. Keyvan-Larijarni, H. and Tannenberg, A. M. (1974). Methanol intoxication: comparison of peritoneal dialysis and hemodialysis treatment. *Arch. Intern. Med.*, **134,** 293–296
81. Jacobsen, D., Jansen, H., Wiik-Larsen, E., Bredesen, J. E. and Halvorsen, S. (1982). Studies on methanol poisoning. *Acta Med. Scand.*, **212,** 5–10
82. Jacobsen, D., Ovrebo, S. and Sejersted, O. M. (1983). Toxokinetics of formate during hemodialysis. *Acta Med. Scand.*, **214,** 409–412
83. McMartin, K. E., Ambre, J. J. and Tephly, T. R. (1980). Methanol poisoning in human subjects. *Am. J. Med.*, **68,** 414–418
84. Vale, J. A., Prior, J. G., O'Hare, J. P., Flanagan, R. J. and Feehally, J. (1982). Treatment of ethylene glycol poisoning with peritoneal dialysis. *Br. Med. J.*, **284,** 557
85. Peterson, C. D., Collins, A. J., Himes, J. M., Bullock, M. L. and Keane, W. F. (1981). Ethylene glycol poisoning. *N. Engl. J. Med.*, **304,** 21–23
86. Rothman, A., Normann, S. A., Manoguerra, A. S., Bastian, J. F. and Griswold, W. R. (1986). Short-term hemodialysis in childhood ethylene glycol poisoning. *J. Pediatr.*, **108,** 153–155

87. Jacobsen, D., Ostby, N. and Bredesen, J. E. (1982). Studies on ethylene glycol poisoning. *Acta Med. Scand.*, **212,** 11–15
88. Jacobsen, D., Ovrebo, S., Ostborg, J. and Sejersted, O. M. (1984). Glycolate causes the acidosis in ethylene glycol poisoning and is effectively removed by hemodialysis. *Acta Med. Scand.*, **216,** 409–416
89. Freireich, A. W., Cinque, T. J., Xanthaky, G. and Landau, D. (1967). Hemodialysis for isopropanol poisoning. *N. Engl. J. Med.*, **277,** 699–700
90. King, H. L., Kent, P. B. and Shires, D. L. (1970). Hemodialysis for isopropyl alcohol poisoning. *J. Am. Med. Assoc.*, **211,** 1855
91. Mecikalski, M. B. and Depner, T. A. (1982). Peritoneal dialysis for isopropanol poisoning. *West J. Med.*, **137,** 322–325
92. Rosansky, S. J. (1982). Isopropyl alcohol poisoning treated with hemodialysis: kinetics of isopropyl alcohol and acetone removal. *Clin. Toxicol.*, **19,** 265–271
93. Dua, S. L. (1974). Peritoneal dialysis for isopropyl alcohol poisoning. *J. Am. Med. Assoc.*, **230,** 235
94. Wilson, J. H. P., Donker, A. J. M., Van Der Hem, G. K. and Wientjes, J. (1971). Peritoneal dialysis for lithium poisoning. *Br. Med. J.*, **2,** 749–750
95. Rosenberg, J., Benowitz, N. L. and Pond, S. (1981). Pharmacokinetics of drug overdose. *Clin. Pharmacokinet.*, **6,** 161–192
96. Clendeninn, N. J., Pond, S. M., Kaysen, G., Barraza, J. J., Farrell, T. and Becker, C. E. (1982). Potential pitfalls in the evaluation of the usefulness of hemodialysis for the removal of lithium. *Clin. Toxicol.*, **19,** 341–352
97. Jaeger, A., Sauder, Ph., Kopferschmitt, J. and Jaegle, M. L. (1985/6). Toxokinetics of lithium intoxication treated by hemodialysis. *Clin. Toxicol.*, **23,** 501–517
98. Von Hartitzsch, B., Hoenich, N. A., Leigh, R. J., Wilkinson, R., Frost, T. H., Weddel, A. and Posen, G. A. (1972). Permanent neurological sequelae despite haemodialysis for lithium intoxication. *Br. Med. J.*, **4,** 757–759
99. Jaeger, A. (1986). Spontaneous toxokinetics of lithium during a therapeutic overdose with renal failure: Response by the authors. *Clin. Toxicol.*, **24,** 265–268
100. Bismuth, C., Baud, F. J., Buneaux, F. and Du Fretay, F. (1986). Spontaneous Toxokinetics of lithium during a therapeutic overdose with renal failure. *Clin. Toxicol.*, **24,** 261–263
101. Miceli, J. N., Clay, B., Fleischmann, L. E., Sarnaik, A. P., Aronow, R. and Done, A. K. (1980). Pharmacokinetics of severe theophylline intoxication managed by peritoneal dialysis. *Dev. Pharmacol. Ther.*, **1,** 16–25
102. Miceli, J. N., Bidani, A. and Aranow, R. (1979). Peritoneal dialysis of theophylline. *Clin. Toxicol.*, **14,** 539–544
103. Brown, G. S., Lohr, T. O., Mayor, G. H., Freitag, J. J., Sanchez, T. V. and Prasad, J. M. (1981). Peritoneal clearance of theophylline. *Am. J. Kidney Dis.*, **1,** 24–26
104. Lee, C. S., Peterson, J. C. and Marbury, T. C. (1983). Comparative pharmacokinetics of theophylline in peritoneal dialysis and hemodialysis. *J. Clin. Pharm.*, **23,** 274–280
105. Woo, O. F., Pond, S. M., Benowitz, N. L. and Olson, K. R. (1984). Benefit of hemoperfusion in acute theophylline intoxication. *Clin. Toxicol.*, **22,** 411–424
106. Levy, G., Gibson, T. P., Whitman, W. and Procknal, J. (1977). Hemodialysis clearance of theophylline. *J. Am. Med. Assoc.*, **237,** 1466–1467

107. Lee, C. S., Marbury, T. C., Perrin, J. H. and Fuller, T. J. (1979). Hemodialysis of theophylline in uremic patients. *J. Clin. Pharm.* **19,** 219–226
108. Yatzidis, H., Voudiclari, S., Oreopoulos, D., Tsaparas, N., Triantaphyllidis, D., Gavras, C. and Stavroulaki, A. (1965). Treatment of severe barbiturate poisoning. *Lancet,* **2,** 216–217
109. Chang, T. M. S., Coffey, J. F., Barre, P., Gonda, A., Dirks, J. H., Levy, M. and Lister, C. (1973). Microcapsule artificial kidney: treatment of patients with acute drug intoxication. *Can. Med. Assoc. J.,* **108,** 429–433
110. Vale, J. A., Rees, A. J., Widdop, B. and Goulding, R. (1975). Use of charcoal haemoperfusion in the management of severely poisoned patients. *Br. Med. J.,* **1,** 5–9
111. Vale, J. A., Thomas, T., Widdop, B. and Goulding, R. (1975). Use of charcoal haemoperfusion in poisoned patients: a review of 20 cases. *Proc. Eur. Soc. Artif. Organ.,* **2,** 239–244
112. Raper, S., Crome, P., Vale, A., Helliwell, M. and Widdop, B. (1982). Experience with activated carbon-bead haemoperfusion columns in the treatment of severe drug intoxication. *Arch. Toxicol.,* **49,** 303–310
113. Rosenbaum, J. L., Kramer, M. S. and Raja, R. (1976). Resin hemoperfusion for acute drug intoxication. *Arch. Intern. Med.,* **136,** 263–266
114. De Groot, G. (1982). Haemoperfusion in clinical toxicology: A pharmacokinetic evaluation. *Published Thesis,* University of Utrecht
115. De Groot, G., Maes, R. A. A. and Van Heyst, A. N. P. (1980). A toxicological evaluation of hemoperfusion using pharmacokinetic principles. In Holmstedt, B., Lauwerys, R., Mercier, M. and Roberfroid, M. (eds.) *Mechanisms of Toxicity and Hazard Evaluation,* pp. 287–395. (Amsterdam: Elsevier/North-Holland)
116. De Groot, G., Maes, R. A. A. and Van Heyst, A. N. P. (1977). The use of haemoperfusion in the elimination of absorbed drug mixtures in acute intoxications. *Neth. J. Med.,* **20,** 142–148
117. Haapanen, E. J. (1982). Hemoperfusion in acute intoxication: clinical experience with 48 cases. *Acta Med. Scand.,* **668** (Suppl.), 76–81
118. Hampel, G., Crome, P., Widdop, B. and Goulding, R. (1980). Experience with fixed-bed charcoal haemoperfusion in the treatment of severe drug intoxication. *Arch. Toxicol.,* **45,** 133–141
119. Gelfand, M. C., Winchester, J. F., Knepshield, J. H., Hanson, K. M., Cohan, S. L., Strauch, B. S., Geoly, K. L., Kennedy, A. C. and Schreiner, G. E. (1977). Treatment of severe drug overdosage with charcoal hemoperfusion. *Trans. Am. Soc. Artif. Organs,* **23,** 599–605
120. Rosenbaum, J. L., Kramer, M. S. and Raja, R. M. (1979). Amberlite hemoperfusion in the treatment of acute drug intoxication. *Int. J. Artif. Organs,* **2,** 316–318
121. Torrente, A., Rumack, B. H., Blair, D. T. and Anderson, R. J. (1979). Fixed-bed uncoated charcoal hemoperfusion in the treatment of intoxications: Animal and patient studies. *Nephron,* **24,** 71–77
122. Barbour, B. H., La Sette, A. M. and Koffler, A. (1976). Fixed-bed charcoal hemoperfusion for the treatment of drug overdose. *Kidney Int.,* **10,** S333–S337
123. Bismuth, C., Fournier, P. E. and Galliot, M. (1981). Biological evaluation of hemoperfusion in acute poisoning. *Clin. Toxicol.,* **18,** 1213–1223
124. Pond, S., Rosenberg, J., Benowitz, N. L., and Takki, S. (1979). Pharmacokinetics of haemoperfusion for drug overdose. *Clin. Pharmacokinet.,* **4,** 329–354

125. Winchester, J. F., Gelfand, M. C. and Tilstone, W. J. (1978). Hemoperfusion in drug intoxication: clinical and laboratory aspects. *Drug Met. Rev.*, **8,** 69–104
126. Benovitz, N., Abolin, C., Tozer, T., Rosenberg, J., Rogers, W., Pond, S., Schoenfeld, P. and Humphreys, M. (1980). Resin hemoperfusion in ethchlorvynol overdose. *Clin. Pharm. Ther.*, **27,** 236–242
127. Nilsson, C., Sterner, G. and Idvall, J. (1984). Charcoal hemoperfusion for treatment of serious carbamazepine poisoning. *Acta Med. Scand.*, **216,** 137–140
128. De Groot, G., Van Heijst, A. N. P. and Maes, R. A. A. (1984). Charcoal hemoperfusion in the treatment of two cases of acute carbamazepine poisoning. *Clin. Toxicol.*, **22,** 349–362
129. Leslie, P. J., Heyworth, R. and Prescott, L. F. (1983). Cardiac complications of carbamazepine: Treatment by haemoperfusion. *Br. Med. J.*, **286,** 1018
130. Heath, A. and Knudsen, K. (1987). Role of extracorporeal drug removal in acute theophylline poisoning: A review. *Med. Toxicol.*, **2,** 294–308
131. Gosselin, B., Mathieu, D., Chopin, C., Wattel, F., Dupuis, B., Haguenoer, J.-M. and Desprey, M. (1980). Acute intoxication with disopyramide: Clinical and experimental study by hemoperfusion on Amberlite XAD-4 resin. *Clin. Toxicol.*, **17,** 439–449
132. Okonek, S. (1980). Intoxication with pyrazolones. *Br. J. Clin. Pharm.*, **10,** 385S–390S
133. Berlinger, W. G., Spector, R., Flanigan, M. J., Johnson, G. F. and Groh, M. R. (1982). Hemoperfusion for phenylbutazone poisoning. *Ann. Intern. Med.*, **96,** 334–335
134. Strong, J. E. Wilson, J., Douglas, J. F. and Coppel, D. L. (1979). Phenylbutazone self-poisoning treated by charcoal haemoperfusion. *Anaesthesia*, **34,** 1038–1040
135. Vale, J. A. (1980). The medical management of acute poisoning: An evaluation of charcoal haemoperfusion. *MD Thesis*, University of London
136. Arieff, A. I. and Friedman, E. A. (1973). Coma following non-narcotic drug overdose: Management of 208 adult patients. *Am. J. Med. Sci.*, **266,** 405–426
137. Salzman, E. W. (1964). Blood platelets and extracorporeal circulation. *Transfusion*, **3,** 274–277
138. De Leval, M., Hill, J. D., Mielke, H., Bramson, M. L., Smith, C. and Gerbode, F. (1972). Platelet kinetics during extracorporeal circulation. *Trans. Am. Soc. Artif. Organs* **28,** 355–358
139. Gimson, A. E. S., Hughes, R. D., Mellon, P. J., Woods, H. F., Langley, P. G., Canalese, J., Williams, R. and Weston, M. J. (1980). Prostacyclin to prevent platelet activation during charcoal haemoperfusion in fulminant hepatic failure. *Lancet*, **1,** 173–175
140. Woods, H. F., Ash, G., Weston, M. J., Bunting, S., Moncada, S. and Vane, J. R. (1978). Prostacyclin can replace heparin in haemodialysis in dogs. *Lancet*, **2,** 1075–1077
141. Vale, A., Meredith, T. and Buckley, B. (1984). Eliminating poisons. *Br. Med. J.*, **289,** 366–369
142. Goodman, L. S. and Gilman, A. G. (1985). In Gilman, A. G., Goodman, L. S., Rall, T. W. and Murad, F. (eds.), *The Pharmacological Basis of Therapeutics*. 7th Edn., p. 1701. (New York: Macmillan)
143. Jacobsen, D., Wiik-Larsen, E., Dahl, T., Enger, E. and Lunde, P. K. M. (1984). Pharmacokinetic evaluation of haemoperfusion in phenobarbital poisoning. *Eur. J. Clin. Pharmacol.*, **26,** 109–112

144. Berlinger, W. G., Spector, R., Goldberg, M. J., Johnson, G. F., Quee, C. K. and Berg, M. J. (1983). Enhancement of theophylline clearance by oral activated charcoal. *Clin. Pharm. Ther.*, **33,** 351–354
145. Mahutte, C. K., True, R. J., Michiels, T. M., Berman, J. M. and Light, R. W. (1983). Increased serum theophylline clearance with orally administered activated charcoal. *Am. Rev. Respir. Dis.*, **128,** 820–822
146. Radomski, L., Park, G. D., Goldberg, M. J., Spector, R., Johnson, G. F. and Quee, C. K. (1984). Model for theophylline overdose treatment with oral activated charcoal. *Clin. Pharm. Ther.*, **35,** 402–408
147. True, R. J., Berman, J. M. and Mahutte, C. K. (1984). Treatment of theophylline toxicity with oral activated charcoal. *Crit. Care Med.*, **12,** 113–114
148. Sessler, C. N., Glauser, F. L. and Cooper, K. R. (1985). Treatment of theophylline toxicity with oral activated charcoal. *Chest*, **87,** 325–329

4
DRUG MONITORING

A.K. SCOTT

Many drugs have a wide therapeutic index and are used with a minimum of supervision. Such an approach is not acceptable for drugs with a narrow therapeutic index and potentially serious side-effects. Also, drugs which are relatively safe in patients with normal renal function may become more difficult to use in the presence of renal failure. These drugs require close monitoring of either their plasma concentration or pharmacodynamic end point.

This review aims to cover aspects of drug monitoring with particular emphasis on the problems in patients with renal disease. Since an understanding of therapeutic drug monitoring requires a basic knowledge of drug disposition and pharmacokinetics, some important aspects of these topics will be discussed first. After consideration of therapeutic drug concentration monitoring, the final section will briefly cover aspects of monitoring drugs by the use of measurable dynamic end points.

EFFECT OF RENAL DISEASE ON DRUG DISPOSITION AND PHARMACOKINETICS

The reduction in clearance of drugs excreted unchanged by the kidney in renal failure is obvious. Renal disease does, however, also have less predictable effects on drug disposition. Changes in drug pharmacokinetics are more likely to be clinically important if the drug has a narrow therapeutic index.

Absorption and bioavailability

Severe renal failure reduces the rate of gastric emptying. This is likely to delay the time taken to reach peak concentration in plasma but does not alter the extent of absorption for most drugs[1]. Such a change is clinically important when a single oral dose is given and a rapid onset of effect is desired, for example, intermittent use of analgesics. The extent of absorption of acid-labile drugs tends to decrease if gastric emptying is delayed. However, this could be offset in renal failure by the rise in pH which occurs due to the buffering of hydrochloric acid by ammonia formed from the increased salivary urea[2]. Further research is necessary to enable a clearer understanding of drug absorption in renal disease.

Bioavailability of a drug is the percentage of an administered dose which reaches the systemic circulation. After oral administration, this depends on the extent of absorption and first-pass metabolism. The effect of renal disease on first-pass metabolism has not been adequately documented. In a study of six patients with chronic renal failure it has been reported that metoclopramide bioavailability was higher and less variable than in normal subjects[3]. This increase in bioavailability was not significant, and was less important than the 70% reduction in total clearance, in explaining the increased incidence of adverse effects of metoclopramide in renal failure. Disopyramide also undergoes extensive first-pass metabolism, but, in three patients with renal failure, plasma concentrations were lower than expected, suggesting the possibility of increased metabolism[4]. This change has been claimed to be due to enzyme induction on the basis of shorter antipyrine half-life and increased D-glucaric acid excretion in patients with renal failure[5]. Enzyme inducers do increase first-pass metabolism and reduce bioavailability of orally administered drugs. However, antipyrine half-life may shorten because of an alteration in volume of distribution, and clearance to individual metabolites is a better test. Urinary D-glucaric acid is likewise not a foolproof measure of enzyme induction, particularly in the presence of renal failure. The effect of renal failure on bioavailability therefore requires further study before general predictions can be made.

Distribution and protein binding

Acidic and neutral drugs tend to bind to albumin, while basic drugs bind predominantly to α_1-acid glycoprotein (AAG). Binding to both of these proteins may be altered in renal disease. Drugs heavily bound to albumin include diazepam, phenytoin, warfarin, sulphonamides, aspirin, other non-steroidal anti-inflammatory drugs and some penicillins. Drugs binding to AAG include disopyramide, lignocaine, propranolol, tricyclic antidepressants and carbamazepine, though these drugs are also partly bound to albumin.

Hypoalbuminaemia from any cause, including nephrotic syndrome, will result in reduced availability of binding sites and reducing binding of phenytoin, diazepam, prednisone and warfarin. For most drugs, the free drug concentration will not show a dramatic change because clearance of the free drug increases if elimination is restricted by protein binding. However, increased toxicity has been reported for phenytoin and warfarin in the presence of hypoalbuminaemia. Drug interactions are also more likely to be clinically important if there are fewer available binding sites. Mutual potentiation of effects has been demonstrated with clofibrate and frusemide used together in nephrotic syndrome[6].

In chronic renal failure, there is reduced binding of drugs to albumin. This is partly accounted for by a reduction in serum albumin concentration. It has been suggested, that, in addition, there is an alteration in the structure of albumin which decreases the affinity for binding drugs. The alteration in albumin structure could be partly due to carbamoylation of lysine residues leading to reduced binding[7]. Carbamoylation occurs due to the spontaneous formation of cyanate from urea. However, the binding capability of plasma can be restored using charcoal treatment at pH 3, and, although carbamoylation does lead to reduced binding *in vitro*, reversal of carbamoylation in uraemic serum does not restore the binding defect[8]. This suggests that the most important cause of the binding defect is the presence of endogenous binding inhibitors. The nature of these inhibitors is not completely understood. Several compounds have been identified as inhibitors of protein binding in uraemia. The responsible metabolites are water soluble organic acids but it is not known whether the problem is due to many weak inhibitors (e.g. hippurates) acting together or to a small number of more potent inhibitors. Indoxyl-3-sulphate and indole-3-acrylic acid are probable contributors to the binding effect. The most potent inhibitor identified is a furanpropionic acid derivative which has recently been shown to be present in uraemic plasma at a concentration which could be important *in vivo*[8]. One of the difficulties in this work is measuring metabolite concentrations present in uraemia so that *in vitro* binding studies can be performed using realistic concentrations of potential binding inhibitors.

Reduced binding has been demonstrated for drugs such as phenytoin, diazepam and warfarin. Reduced binding *per se* does not necessarily lead to altered drug effect as the free drug concentration may be unchanged. However, knowledge of reduced binding is very important in the interpretation of drug concentrations during therapeutic drug monitoring (TDM). Most laboratories report concentrations of total drug (bound + free) and rely on a reasonably constant relationship between free and total drug. If this relationship is disturbed, as in renal failure, the total concentration will not relate well to the free drug concentration. The 'therapeutic range' needs to be adjusted downwards to compensate for this change. In addition, the response to the drug may alter in the presence of disease and further complicate the process of TDM.

More recently, it has been recognized that AAG concentration is increased, with an increase in binding of basic drugs, such as lignocaine, in renal failure. Endogenous binding inhibitors, therefore, do not appear to influence binding to AAG. This will again lead to difficulty in interpreting drug concentrations but with a need for upward adjustment of the therapeutic range. Drugs affected are carbamazepine and lignocaine.

Reduction in protein binding of heavily bound drugs tends to lead to an increase in volume of distribution (Vd). This has been shown for phenytoin, diazepam and warfarin. The chief significance of this observation is that, assuming there is no change in drug clearance (Cl), the elimination half-life ($t_{\frac{1}{2}}$) should be prolonged ($t_{\frac{1}{2}} = 0.693 \times \mathrm{Vd/Cl}$). Any increase in clearance may offset the effect of the increased volume of distribution on half-life but this requires to be studied for individual drugs. Half-life is therefore not a useful guide for predicting changes in maintenance dose in renal failure. However, if half-life is prolonged, it may be necessary to increase the dosing interval.

Metabolism

It is conventionally recommended that patients with renal failure should be prescribed drugs eliminated by hepatic metabolism where possible. The effect of renal disease on drug metabolism is not well documented and it cannot be assumed that there is no such effect. The reports which are available do not show a consistent pattern. As discussed above, the metabolism of antipyrine and disopyramide has been claimed to be increased in renal failure. However, in another study using antipyrine given intravenously, there was a reduction in half-life with no change in volume of distribution in the presence of renal failure. Also, in patients with nephrotic syndrome and no renal failure, antipyrine kinetics were similar to normal controls. It has been suggested that phenytoin metabolism is accelerated in uraemia and that this cannot be totally accounted for by the reduced protein binding[9]. In contrast, clearance of unbound diazepam is not significantly altered in end-stage renal failure[10] and dihydrocodeine clearance is reduced in renal failure though it is not clear if this is due to reduced hepatic elimination[11].

Although renal excretion of unchanged drug is not a major route of elimination for most drugs, the kidney is very important for the excretion of drug metabolites, which are more water soluble than the parent drug. The importance of drug metabolites in renal failure has been reviewed[12] with four main patterns considered likely to cause problems:

(1) The accumulation of active metabolites (e.g. allopurinol, clofibrate, pethidine) may result in potentiation of the drug effect, or, in some cases, toxicity.
(2) Inactive metabolites may interfere with the kinetics of the parent drug by competing for binding sites or perhaps inhibiting further metabolism.
(3) Glucuronides may be deconjugated to regenerate active drug.
(4) Results from several studies are difficult to interpret because assay methods do not reliably distinguish between parent drug and metabolites. A recent example of this is the use of a specific HPLC assay for morphine to demonstrate that morphine-6-glucuronide, but not morphine, accumulates in renal failure[13]. Morphine-6-glucuronide may be an active metabolite.

The kidney itself may have an important role in drug metabolism. This may result in the local production of toxic metabolites which result in renal damage (e.g. paracetamol) or be simply one of the extrahepatic sites of drug metabolism with the production of inactive compounds.

Excretion

Reduced elimination of unchanged drug is clearly to be expected in renal failure. Where renal elimination is the only significant route (atenolol, digoxin, gentamicin), drug clearance will fall in the presence of renal failure and drug maintenance dosage will need to be reduced. Renal failure may also be important for drugs which are partly metabolized and each drug needs to be considered individually. Elimination by glomerular filtration (e.g. digoxin, atenolol) and tubular secretion (e.g. penicillins, frusemide, salicylates) are both affected. Individual drugs will be considered in more detail below.

EFFECT OF RENAL DISEASE ON DRUG PHARMACODYNAMICS

There is much less information on the effect of renal disease on drug pharmacodynamics. Expression of a drug effect usually involves the interaction of the drug with its receptors, a series of intermediate reactions and the final clinical effect. Since the intermediate pathways are poorly understood it is clearly difficult to determine the mechanism of any alterations in response which occur in renal failure. As discussed above, binding of drugs to protein is altered in renal failure. It is therefore possible that drug receptor proteins could have an altered configuration in uraemia which could increase or decrease the response to a given drug concentration. Also accumulation of endogenous compounds might reduce drug binding to receptors.

More detailed investigation of drug kinetics in renal failure will be necessary before alterations in receptor sensitivity can be adequately studied. A recent example of this is the investigation of the increase in sensitivity to opiates in renal failure. Application of modern methodology to measure parent drug and active metabolite for morphine suggests that the problem is probably a kinetic one due to reduced excretion of morphine-6-glucuronide[13]. Patients with renal failure are also more sensitive to other sedative drugs but whether all can be explained on a kinetic rather than dynamic mechanism remains to be determined.

THERAPEUTIC DRUG MONITORING

Therapeutic drug monitoring (TDM) is the measurement of drug concentrations in a suitable body fluid (usually serum or plasma) to allow adjustment of dose, either to reduce toxicity or improve efficacy or both. In many hospitals, the drug concentration measurement is returned to the clinician with no attempt to advise on dose adjustment. However, in some centres, advice is given on suitable dose adjustments using computer-based predictive equations where appropriate. Whether the dose is adjusted by the clinician alone or with the advice from laboratory-based colleagues, it is essential that the prescriber has a knowledge of how concomitant disease affects the interpretation of the results.

It is possible to measure blood concentrations of all drugs but there is benefit from monitoring levels in only a small number of situations. For a drug to be a suitable candidate for TDM, it should satisfy most of the following criteria:

(1) The effective therapeutic range should be clearly defined and adequately validated in controlled clinical trials.

The therapeutic range for drugs currently considered for TDM is unfortunately not well defined for several drugs. For example, there is debate about the range for theophylline and the upper limit for valproate. In contrast, the range for phenytoin has been well documented, though concentrations must still be interpreted with respect to all available clinical information.

(2) There is no precise dynamic end point which can be measured to assess drug reaction.

TDM only allows correction for interindividual variation in pharmacokinetic parameters. It does not allow for variation in receptor sensitivity and response to the interaction of drug with receptor.

If a pharmacodynamic end point (e.g. prothrombin time for warfarin; pulse rate for β-blockers) is available, then it should be used in preference to TDM.

(3) Wide interindividual variation in dose required to produce a desired steady-state drug concentration.

This makes it difficult to predict the required dose for an individual patient. TDM is not very useful if the interindividual variation is mainly due to receptor sensitivity rather than kinetics as noted above.

(4) A relationship between plasma drug or active metabolite concentration and the clinical response exists.

For most drugs this relationship is poorly defined. If there is a good correlation between concentration and response, it suggests that there is little interindividual variation in receptor sensitivity.

(5) A low therapeutic index with potentially serious dose-related adverse effects.

TDM will not help to reduce non-dose-related toxicity. If the important side-effects are not dose related, there is little benefit from monitoring concentrations.

(6) The level at which dose-related side-effects are likely to occur should be known.

TDM is particularly important if the symptoms of drug toxicity resemble the symptoms of the underlying disease, as clinical judgement would clearly be unreliable in that situation.

(7) A validated assay method must be available for measurement of the active moiety – parent drug, metabolite or both.

The method must be suitable for routine use with no interference from other drugs or endogenous compounds. Ideally, it would be better to measure the free drug concentration rather than total drug. However, in practice, it is more difficult and more expensive to measure free drug concentration on a routine basis.

Patients with renal disease are at greater risk of adverse drug effects and some drugs suitable for TDM are predominantly excreted unchanged by the kidney. TDM is therefore likely to be of considerable benefit in patient with renal failure. There are, however, additional problems in the use of TDM in renal disease:

(1) The optimum therapeutic range in renal disease may be different from that in patients with normal renal function. The effects of renal failure on receptor sensitivity are not well established. Some drugs clearly have an enhanced effect in renal failure but it is often difficult to separate the effect of kinetic changes from true changes in the dynamic response. Adenosine triphosphatases (ATPase) are involved in the action of digoxin and perhaps also of the anticonvulsants. Renal failure alters the concentration of ions (sodium, potassium, magnesium) which affect ATPase activity. It is also possible that the enzyme structure is altered in renal disease. Response may therefore be altered and could vary from day to day depending on the effects of other drug treatment (e.g. diuretics) or the time in relation to dialysis. At present, no clear guidelines can be given to allow for this problem, except that extra care is necessary to detect adverse effects even if the blood concentration is not excessive. Increased vigilance is necessary to ensure that the expected clinical response is obtained.

(2) Total drug concentration is measured in most laboratories but pharmacological effect and adverse effects are related to free drug concentration. TDM works in most situations because there is a reasonably close relationship between free and total drug concentrations.

This is not true in the presence of renal failure. Drug binding to albumin is reduced in the presence of renal failure while binding to AAG tends to increase. The mechanisms for this have been discussed above. If drugs are heavily protein bound, even small changes in binding can result in large changes in the free fraction. For example, if drug A is normally 95% bound, the free fraction is 5%. If, however, the bound fraction falls to 90%, the free fraction doubles to 10%. Knowledge of this problem is very important when interpreting drug concentrations, because, if attempts are made to achieve the usual therapeutic range, the free concentration could be double the expected concentration for drug A. It is necessary to aim for a lower target range in the presence of renal failure if TDM is undertaken for drugs binding heavily to albumin. Both phenytoin and sodium valproate are extensively bound to albumin.

Less is known about alterations in the therapeutic range of basic drugs which bind mainly to AAG. Carbamazepine is such a drug and its binding would be expected to increase in the presence of renal failure. Interpretation of carbamazepine concentrations is further complicated by the presence of a metabolite (carbamazepine-10,11-epoxide) which is responsible for around 50% of the total anti-convulsant activity. In this situation, it is necessary to measure free concentration of parent drug and metabolite. For carbamezepine, it is technically easier to measure salivary concentrations which give a reliable prediction of free concentration in plasma[14].

Therapeutic drug monitoring is generally available for the drugs shown in Table 4.1. In addition, monitoring is available for a small number of other drugs (e.g. lignocaine, antidepressants) in some centres. Drug concentration measurement is undertaken following deliberate or accidental overdosage with a wide variety of drugs (e.g. aspirin, paracetamol, benzodiazepines, alcohol) and the effects of renal disease on these measurements will also be discussed. Finally, drug concentrations are sometimes measured to assess patient compliance, for example, warfarin when the diagnosis is between non-compliance and warfarin resistance.

TABLE 4.1 Drugs for which a therapeutic drug monitoring service is generally available

Anticonvulsants –	phenytoin
	carbamazepine
	sodium valproate
	phenobarbitone
	primidone
	ethosuximide
Digoxin	
Gentamicin	
Lithium	
Theophylline	

When the drugs listed in Table 4.1 are considered, most are either predominantly excreted unchanged by the kidneys (digoxin, gentamicin, lithium) or are extensively protein bound (phenytoin, carbamazepine, valproate). Renal disease affects both of these processes.

Assay methods

A detailed description of assay methods used in TDM is beyond the scope of this review. Older colorimetric methods should not be used for routine measurements except following deliberate or accidental overdose when a rapid result is essential. TDM laboratories should now use either chromatography (usually HPLC) or specific antibody-based methods (e.g. enzyme multiplied immunotechnique – EMIT; radioimmunoassay – RIA). Prescribers cannot be expected to know which drugs may co-elute with the drug being measured by HPLC or those which cross react with the antibody used in EMIT or RIA methods. Prescribers should list other drug therapy and disease states on the request form so that the laboratory staff can decide if their assay technique is suitable for the individual patient.

New methods suitable for routine service use need to be developed to measure concentration of free drug and active metabolites for some drugs. These will be discussed below.

Individual drugs

Digoxin

Digoxin is used for two main indications – atrial flutter/fibrillation and cardiac failure. When used for the treatment of atrial fibrillation, the aim is to control the ventricular rate. In this situation, there is a readily available (though not infallible) dynamic end point in that the heart rate can be measured by auscultation and the pulse deficit noted. The dose of digoxin can be titrated against the heart rate. TDM, therefore, has limited application but is of some value in reducing toxicity and assessing patient compliance.

In cardiac failure, there is no easily measurable end point for use at the bedside. The clinical benefit may be delayed and is often difficult to assess because of the effects of other drugs (e.g. diuretics). TDM is therefore important to ensure that the serum digoxin concentration is within the therapeutic range (0.8–2.0 μg/ml). There is no benefit in continuing therapy with an ineffective dose or a dose likely to lead to significant adverse effects.

The maintenance dose of digoxin will be lower in the presence of renal failure because of reduced renal clearance. Digoxin is mainly excreted by glomerular filtration and its clearance correlated closely with creatinine clearance. A small proportion undergoes tubular secretion and reabsorption. In most patients, less than 20% of a dose of digoxin is metabolized. However, a small number of patients exhibit more extensive metabolism of digoxin to an inactive metabolite (dihydrodigoxin). These patients are less likely to show significant accumulation of digoxin if they develop renal failure. There is interindividual variation in dose requirements for any given level of renal function and an overlap of the dose ranges in normals compared with patients with impaired renal function.

Since digoxin has a long half-life (36 h), which is prolonged in renal failure (over 100 h in severe disease), it is necessary to give a loading dose in most patients. The loading dose of a drug depends on the volume of distribution rather than clearance. Volume of distribution of digoxin is reduced by around 50% in renal failure, though the extent is variable and depends partly on the degree of renal impairment. In practice, the loading dose also depends on weight, age and sex and there is overlap between normals and patients with renal failure. Loading doses are now generally given in divided doses 6–8 h apart. The initial dose may be 250 or 500 μg depending on the size of the patient. Further 250 μg doses can then be given six hourly while the patient is monitored for signs of beneficial effect and toxicity. Most patients will require between 500 μg and 1.5 mg. This approach is suitable for patients with normal renal function and those with renal impairment. Patients with renal failure will tend to need smaller loading doses on average but these cannot be easily predicted on an individual basis. It is usually important to achieve the therapeutic effect within a few hours and then monitor the response and serum concentration to ensure the correct maintenance dose for the degree of renal impairment.

In view of digoxin's reputation as a toxic drug, considerable effort has been made to attempt to predict digoxin dose requirements for individual patients[15,16]. The most simple method for use at the bedside is a nomogram for prediction of both loading and maintenance dose based on the patient's weight, sex and renal function (serum creatinine or creatinine clearance). Alternatively there are equations available which allow dose predictions similar to the nomogram, but many clinicians lack enthusiasm for using mathematics in practice. Finally, several computer programs have been developed to simplify dose prediction. The main drawback is the lack of immediate access to computers in most hospitals, though this is likely to change over the next decade.

Before embarking on a move away from traditional intuitive methods for digoxin dose determination, clinicians need to know whether new methods lead to improvement in patient care. Several studies have evaluated equations and computer programs against the performance of clinicians. The overall impression is that there is little difference in outcome when an experienced clinician is compared with the predictive methods. This is not entirely surprising, because no allowance has been made for variation in receptor sensitivity and there is very little flexibility in the strength of digoxin tablets which can be administered. If the predictive methods calculate that the maintenance dose should be 235 μg, this may be more accurate than the clinician's guess of 250 μg, but the dose given will still need to be 250 μg because of tablet availability. An average daily dose of 232 μg could be achieved by giving 250 μg daily for six days and 125 μg each Sunday. However, variations from standard, fixed daily doses tend to lead to problems with reduced patient compliance. This is particularly true in the elderly and most digoxin prescriptions are for patients over 60 years old.

Predictive methods, therefore, are of little benefit to the experienced clinician who remembers to adjust the dose with respect to individual patient factors (renal function, hypokalaemia, age, thyroid disease) known to affect digoxin kinetics and response. Less experienced prescribers should consider the use of the nomogram in conjunction with measurements of digoxin concentration until good control is established. Excessive blood concentration monitoring is not necessary. It has been reported that optimum benefit is obtained from two concentration measurements with no additional benefit from further samples. The two measurements should be taken 1–2 weeks apart. Such an approach is useful to ensure reduced digoxin toxicity, adequate concentration for therapeutic effect in cardiac failure, and for the education of the clinician.

When a sample for digoxin or other drug measurement is sent to the laboratory, it is important that all relevant information is included on the request form, particularly if the laboratory will suggest alterations in dose.

Such information includes:

(1) Adequate identification of sample and patient.
(2) Patient details – age, sex, weight, renal function.
(3) Other disease.
(4) Other drug therapy.
(5) Time of sample.
(6) Time of last dose.
(7) Dose and frequency of administration.

When collecting blood for measurement of digoxin concentration, it is essential to take the sample at least 6 h after the last dose. Measurements within the distribution phase (1–5 h) do not accurately reflect steady-state concentration.

Digoxin is one of the main drugs responsible for serious adverse effects and features prominantly in studies into the high incidence (5–10%) of adverse drug effects in medical emergency admissions. A recent survey of digoxin concentrations found that only 35% were within the therapeutic range while 37% were above it[17]. After issue of a laboratory report with advice on the necessary dose alterations, the number within the therapeutic range improved to 66% with a fall to 15% above the range. Half of the patients with elevated serum concentrations were still receiving double the recommended dose. This study clearly shows that improvement is possible with a laboratory reporting system to give advice on dose changes. Such advice is likely to be even more relevant for patients with renal impairment.

Gentamicin

Gentamicin is a potentially toxic aminoglycoside antibiotic with a narrow therapeutic index. It is mainly used for the treatment of infection due to Gram-negative bacilli. There is no measurable end point which allows control of drug dosage. Gentamicin is therefore generally considered to be a suitable candidate for TDM. This is particularly important in renal failure for two reasons. Firstly, gentamicin is excreted almost entirely in the unchanged form by glomerular filtration. Secondly, nephrotoxicity is one of the principal adverse effects. Gentamicin accumulates in proximal renal tubular cells and causes progressive tubular damage. This is reversible if the drug is stopped at an early stage. If gentamicin is continued, further renal impairment develops, leading to greater accumulation of drug and enhanced toxicity.

There is little hard evidence on which to base a therapeutic range for gentamicin[18]. It is usually recommended that both peak and trough concentrations should be measured. To be effective, antibiotics need to be administered in doses which will give a local concentration which is higher than the minimum concentration necessary to inhibit bacterial growth (MIC). The MIC varies with different organisms and it is not usually possible to measure the antibiotic concentration at the site of infection. However, the serum drug concentration is in equilibrium with the concentration in infected tissue and is a useful guide in avoiding subtherapeutic drug administration. The peak concentration of gentamicin for optimum response appears to be around 5–10 μg/ml except in neutropaenic patients who respond better when the level is above 10 μg/ml. In patients with normal host defences, it is considered that intermittent therapy is satisfactory with trough levels around 1–2 μg/ml.

The principal side-effects of gentamicin – nephrotoxicity and ototoxicity – are dose related. Up to 10% of patients on gentamicin suffer mild renal damage and 2% have severe renal impairment. There is debate as to whether renal damage is due to very high peak levels or insufficiently low trough levels, or a combination of both. Trough levels of greater than 4 μg/ml are associated with a high incidence (100% in some studies) of nephrotoxicity. However, it is difficult to separate cause and effect in this situation, as many patients with elevated trough concentrations have abnormal renal function before gentamicin is administered. The elevated trough concentrations are due to reduced gentamicin clearance. High peak levels do not show a good correlation with nephrotoxicity and are not influenced by renal failure unless accumulation occurs because of frequent dosing.

Nephrotoxicity is more common in the presence of other potentially nephrotoxic drugs and is increased by diuretics such as frusemide. Extra care is therefore necessary if such drugs are given concomitantly. In particular, frusemide in high doses is commonly prescribed in renal failure.

As with nephrotoxicity, eighth nerve damage occurs in up to 10% of patients given gentamicin, and more severe damage causing symptoms occurs in around 2%. This is often permanent. Ototoxicity is more likely in patients with renal disease. In one study, 64% of patients with ototoxicity had pre-existing renal impairment. This confirms the necessity for close control of gentamicin dosing in patients with renal failure. As with nephrotoxicity, the evidence for the relative importance of peak and trough levels is inconclusive. Animal studies suggest that high peaks are important, but, in man, it is difficult to separate peak from trough effects. There is some evidence that peak concentrations around 10 μg/ml, which is at the upper end of the reported concentration range necessary for therapeutic effect, can cause damage. Patients with high trough concentrations are certainly at increased risk of eighth nerve damage. However, as with nephrotoxicity, high trough levels are associated with reduced renal clearance of gentamicin. It is therefore not clear whether peak and trough levels *per se* are important, or whether it is the total exposure to drug as measured by the area under the concentration–time curve. Patients with high trough concentrations inevitably have high total exposure.

Although the evidence is inconclusive, it is important to have practical target peak and trough concentrations. Based on available evidence, the peak concentration should be 8–10 μg/ml to achieve a useful effect with low risk of toxicity. Trough concentrations should be around 2 μg/ml. In practice, it is not always easy to achieve this ideal as alterations in both total dose and dosing interval will be necessary in patients with renal failure. If the trough level is above 4 μg/ml, the dosing interval should be increased, while high peak levels are avoided by reducing the amount of drug given. In patients with normal renal function, one set of peak and trough measurements is often sufficient to achieve satisfactory concentrations. However, in renal failure, repeated measurements are necessary to achieve the desired drug profile. In this situation, it is essential to have a rapid result from the laboratory so that appropriate adjustments can be made before the next dose is given.

The difficulty in achieving satisfactory drug concentrations in individual patients has resulted, as for digoxin, in attempts to develop nomograms and equations for use either at the bedside or in the laboratory[16]. Prediction of the initial dose from knowledge of the patient's renal function, weight, age and sex has been attempted using techniques ranging from a simple nomogram to the use of a mainframe computer. These have not been extensively evaluated and are not sufficiently accurate to allow the use of gentamicin without further concentration measurements. The presence of additional information in the form of actual peak and trough concentrations following a known dose of gentamicin improves the ability of computer programs to predict accurate dose changes. Several schemes for dose adjustment in this way are already in use but require evaluation of their benefit. In view of the nature of gentamicin toxicity, it should be easier to demonstrate benefit than has been the case for digoxin.

Careful monitoring is also necessary for patients on dialysis. Gentamicin is readily cleared from the blood during haemodialysis and care is necessary to adequately supplement the dose of gentamicin during periods of dialysis. The clearance of gentamicin during peritoneal dialysis is poor and less predictable but supplementation may be necessary in some patients. This can only be determined on an individual basis by monitoring gentamicin concentrations.

A typical starting dose in adults should be 80 mg eight hourly. In patients with normal renal function, this may need to be altered following serum concentration measurement, particularly to avoid underdosing. In patients with creatinine clearance values greater than 50 ml/min, the initial dose should be unchanged but the dosing interval could be increased to 12 hourly. With more severe failure (creatinine clearance 10–50 ml/min), a suitable regime is 80 mg initially then 50 mg 12 hourly. When creatinine clearance is less than 10 ml/min, 80 mg loading dose could be followed by 30 mg daily. It is important to emphasize again that such doses are only a guide and it is essential to monitor concentrations both to reduce the incidence of toxicity and to ensure that effective serum concentrations have been achieved.

Lithium

Lithium is used in the treatment of manic depression to prevent mood swings. It has a narrow therapeutic range (0.8–1.2 mmol/L) with serious dose-related adverse effects which occur in most patients just above the upper end of the therapeutic range. Since it is difficult to objectively assess a patient's mood and, also, there is a delay in response to lithium, there is no useful dynamic end point. Lithium is therefore a suitable candidate for TDM.

Lithium is handled by the body in the same way as sodium. It is free in solution and distributes throughout the body water. Elimination is mainly by renal excretion of unchanged drug. Lithium clearance depends on renal function as well as on sodium balance and urine volume. Patients who are sodium depleted conserve sodium by reducing its loss in the urine. When this occurs, lithium excretion is also reduced. In addition, diuretics inhibit lithium excretion and cause a clinically important rise in serum concentrations. This is more marked with thiazide diuretics.

There is less information on monitoring lithium than is available for digoxin and gentamicin. As with digoxin there is variation in bioavailability with different products. The same brand should therefore be used throughout treatment. Also, the timing of the sample is crucial and should be twelve hours post dose if twice-daily dosing is used, or between 12 and 24 hours post dose for once-daily administration. The elimination half-life is 14–28 h. It will, therefore, take 4–5 days to achieve steady-state concentrations.

If creatinine clearance is greater than 50 ml/min, lithium carbonate should be started in a dose of 400 mg daily and blood levels checked 12 hours after the fifth dose. Daily dose requirements can then be reassessed if the serum concentration is outside the therapeutic range. Concentration increases linearly with respect to dose; therefore, dose adjustment is relatively straightforward if the blood sample has been collected at the correct time. Dose reductions should be made for patients with significant renal failure if it is felt that the benefits of lithium treatment outweigh the increased risk in renal disease. The initial dose should still be 400 mg for the first day because the longer half-life in renal failure would mean a long time to reach steady state. However, from day 2–5, 200 mg daily could be given if the creatinine clearance is 10–50 ml/min and 100 mg daily if creatinine clearance is less than 10 ml/min.

It is essential not to delay checking serum concentration beyond seven days from starting therapy if side-effects are to be avoided. Most patients will not develop adverse effects until a concentration of 1.5 mmol/L is reached but some are more sensitive to the drug. Although there is no satisfactory dynamic end point for assessing the therapeutic efficacy, we can monitor end points for toxicity. It is important to look for finger tremor and nystagmus as well as questioning the patient regarding gastrointestinal symptoms, thirst and polyuria. With long-term use, lithium may cause renal damage and renal function should also be monitored. Undetected development of renal failure will lead to lithium toxicity because of reduced drug clearance.

Nomograms have not been found to be useful for lithium. Toxicity is best avoided by careful concentration monitoring, adjusting the dose in the presence of renal failure and when diuretics are prescribed. Lithium is removed from the blood by dialysis and particular care is required to keep such patients within the therapeutic range.

Finally, a common mistake is to send a sample for plasma lithium measurement in a tube anticoagulated with lithium–heparin. It will avoid the need for a second sample if a plain tube is used for serum measurements.

Anticonvulsant Therapy

Phenytoin

Phenytoin is one of the most commonly used drugs in the treatment of epilepsy. Prior to the introduction of drug concentration measurement, many patients with epilepsy were treated with multiple drug therapy. Drug monitoring has played a major part in the move to ensure adequate therapy with a single anticonvulsant wherever possible. Most patients are now treated with only one or two drugs. Phenytoin is a good candidate for therapeutic drug monitoring. There is wide interindividual variation in phenytoin pharmacokinetics with a non-linear relationship between dose and plasma concentration. Phenytoin has a narrow therapeutic index with definite dose-related toxicity. The therapeutic range (10–20 mg/L) has been well documented in controlled studies. Most of the patients in the studies had moderate to severe disease and it is possible that patients with mild disease may be controlled at slightly lower concentrations. The dynamic end point (control of seizures) is difficult to use as a method of dose titration unless the seizures are very frequent. However, it is always important to treat the patient's problem, and, if total control of seizures is obtained at a concentration below the therapeutic range, then it is not necessary to adjust the dose.

Phenytoin is an interesting drug to study because of the way it is handled by the body. However, the interindividual variation in its pharmacokinetic parameters make it a difficult drug to use unless the prescriber has a thorough understanding of drug disposition. Phenytoin absorption is dependent on the formulation used, as the excipient in the tablet is important in determining phenytoin bioavailability. It is therefore essential to use the same formulation throughout treatment. If there are compelling reasons for changing to a different brand, the plasma concentrations must be monitored. Renal disease appears to have little effect on phenytoin absorption.

Phenytoin is normally around 90% bound to albumin in plasma. As has been discussed above, renal failure results in reduced protein binding, due mainly to the accumulation of endogenous binding inhibitors which are normally excreted in the urine. In nephrotic syndrome, phenytoin protein binding is reduced because of low serum albumin concentrations even in the absence of renal failure. Phenytoin half-life depends on the dose given. It has been reported that the half-life is reduced in renal failure. Phenytoin may have to be given more frequently to avoid excessive swings in blood concentration. However, there are no predictable changes in dose requirements in renal failure and careful titration is necessary on an individual patient basis. When TDM is undertaken to check that the concentration achieved following dose alteration is within the target range, it is important to allow four half-life times before taking the blood sample.

The most important problem in TDM for phenytoin in the presence of renal impairment is interpretation of the result obtained with reference to the standard therapeutic range. Most laboratories measure total phenytoin concentration with a therapeutic range of 10–20 mg/L. Free drug is considered to be the active moiety and it is assumed that there is close correlation between free and total drug concentration. However, in renal failure, we know that there is reduced protein binding and care must be taken to avoid overdosing. If the dose of phenytoin is adjusted to aim for a total concentration within the usual target range, the higher percentage of free drug will result in an increase in the actual free drug concentration, which may fall into the toxic range. Toxicity can usually be avoided if phenytoin concentrations are kept within the lower half (10–15 ml/L) of the target range. In many patients, lower total concentrations will be adequate. This problem can be overcome by measuring free phenytoin concentration directly but most laboratories do not yet offer this facility.

Alteration of phenytoin dose also causes problems for the unwary. Phenytoin is one of the few drugs for which the enzymes responsible for metabolism in the liver become saturated within the therapeutic dose range. All drug-metabolizing enzymes have limited capacity and most will become saturated if a large enough overdose is taken. However, the enzymes responsible for phenytoin metabolism have relatively low capacity which tends to reach the point of saturation with a daily intake of 200–300 mg. Up to the point of saturation, there is a linear relationship between dose and plasma concentration. Above this point, metabolism becomes zero order – the amount of drug metabolized is constant per unit of time irrespective of the drug concentration. Plasma concentrations therefore rise much more rapidly than might be expected for a given dose increase[19]. Above a dose of 300 mg daily, increases in dose must be in small increments. Phenytoin is available in 25 and 50 mg doses so that this can be achieved.

Not surprisingly, the difficulties in using phenytoin have led to attempts to develop methods of predicting individual dose requirements and dose adjustments. There are no reliable methods of predicting an individual's initial dose of phenytoin. As a result, the initial dose is fixed for most patients. Two schools of thought exist. One is that the initial daily dose should be 200 mg with increases as necessary. The advantage of this regime is that dose-related toxicity is very unlikely to occur. However, the disadvantage is that most patients will not be adequately controlled with the initial dose used. There is recent evidence that it is important to achieve early control of seizures in order to obtain the best degree of long-term control. The alternative approach is to give an initial dose of 300 mg daily (200 mg at night, 100 mg in the morning) and adjust the dose as required. The advantage here is of earlier control of seizures in more patients. The disadvantage is that some patients have a genetically-controlled defect in phenytoin metabolism and will develop potentially toxic phenytoin concentrations even with this low dose. The latter approach is favoured by the author and toxic effects can usually be avoided if a sample is taken for TDM soon after reaching steady-state concentration (about 1 week after commencing therapy).

Several methods have been developed for predicting dose adjustments of phenytoin following the initiation of treatment. As with digoxin, these have taken the form of equations, nomograms and computer programs. Computer-based methods may be satisfactory if the hardware is already available, but, for routine clinical use at the bedside, there is a nomogram available which is easy to use[20]. This nomogram requires a knowledge of the initial or previous dose given and a measure of the steady-state plasma concentration. The dose change necessary to achieve a target concentration, say 15 mg/ml, is simply obtained by drawing two lines on a graph. Experienced and regular prescribers of phenytoin soon learn the dose changes necessary for a given plasma concentration. However, for infrequent users of phenytoin, the nomogram is a valuable tool for avoiding both excessively long periods of underdosing and dose-related toxicity. A repeat serum phenytoin measurement should be made after dose adjustment to check that the desired concentration has been achieved.

In the presence of renal failure, the nomogram could still be used, though it has not been evaluated in that situation. The plasma concentration measured following the initial dose allows for the effect of disease on drug kinetics. However, as discussed above, it is important to allow adequate time to reach steady state before taking the plasma sample for TDM. Also the target total phenytoin concentration should be lowered to allow for the reduced protein binding.

Whether in the presence of normal renal function or renal failure, it is essential to ensure that the patient has been taking the medication as prescribed. Non-compliance with treatment would lead to the predicted dose being too large. It is also important to ensure that the plasma sample is taken in the excretion phase of phenytoin dosing and not too close to the last dose taken.

Carbamazepine
Like phenytoin, carbamazepine is a frequently used potent anticonvulsant. The value of therapeutic drug monitoring for carbamazepine is, however, less clearly defined. The therapeutic range for carbamazepine has not been as fully evaluated as that for phenytoin and there are specific problems in undertaking TDM for carbamazepine.

Carbamazepine is a heavily protein-bound drug but, unlike phenytoin, it binds to both albumin and α_1-acid glycoprotein. The binding to albumin may be reduced in renal failure. However, AAG concentration increases in renal failure with an increase in carbamazepine binding. In addition, blood AAG concentrations show considerable day-to-day variation. This makes it impossible to assume a good relationship between total and free drug concentrations. Carbamazepine is mainly metabolized to carbamazepine 10,11-epoxide which is responsible for about 50% of the total anticonvulsant activity. Carbamazepine concentrations are not significantly altered in renal failure but the metabolite elimination is reduced. Clearly, measurement of total plasma carbamazepine concentration can be of little help in optimizing carbamazepine dose in patients with normal renal function and is of no real value in the presence of renal failure.

It is essential to monitor free concentration of both parent drug and its epoxide metabolite in patients with renal failure. This is technically difficult and most laboratories measure saliva concentrations of drug and metabolite because this approximates to the free concentration in plasma.

Sodium valproate
For the treatment of major seizures, valproate is now considered to be as effective as phenytoin or carbamazepine.

There is considerable debate as to the value of TDM for treatment of epilepsy with sodium valproate. The chief concern is with the upper end of the therapeutic range. Acute dose-related toxicity is less of a problem with valproate than with phenytoin or carbamazepine. There is, therefore, an argument for raising the upper end of the target range

(100 mg/L). TDM has some value in ensuring that the patient is compliant with therapy and that the trough plasma concentration is above the lower end of the target range (50 mg/L). However, if a patient fails to achieve an adequate response at a concentration within the therapeutic range, there is a strong case for increasing the dose if there are good reasons why more effective drugs cannot be used. Clearly, if higher doses are used, it is essential that the patient is closely monitored for early signs of drug toxicity.

In the presence of renal failure, the main difficulty is similar to that for phenytoin. Valproate is extensively protein bound (90%) to albumin and the bound fraction decreases in the presence of endogenous binding inhibitors. Low total concentrations do not necessarily mean inadequate concentration of free drug.

Other anticonvulsants

The therapeutic ranges of other anticonvulsants have not been fully evaluated and are less clearly defined. TDM is at least of value in assessing compliance and ensuring that subtherapeutic doses are avoided in the presence of inadequate seizure control. There are few additional problems when monitoring in the presence of renal failure.

Phenobarbitone is 25–50% excreted unchanged depending on urinary pH. In alkaline urine, the amount excreted by the kidneys increases. Phenobarbitone is not extensively protein bound (around 50%) so that binding changes are less important. In severe renal impairment, the dose should be reduced to compensate for reduced renal excretion. Primidone is also not extensively protein bound but the half-life is increased in renal failure and the dosing interval may need to be lengthened.

Ethosuximide is only 10% protein bound. Elimination is mainly by hepatic metabolism and dose reduction is only necessary in severe renal failure when creatinine clearance is less than 10 ml/min.

Clonazepam may be measured in some laboratories. There is no evidence of benefit from TDM and no particular kinetic problems in renal failure. However, excess sedation may occur, perhaps due to altered receptor function in end-stage renal disease. Should this occur the dose must be reduced.

Theophylline

Theophylline is a bronchodilator with a narrow therapeutic index. There is wide interindividual variation in its pharmacokinetics, and, like phenytoin, there is evidence of saturation kinetics occurring within the normal therapeutic dose range. Side-effects are predominantly dose related and some are potentially serious. In the presence of concomitant renal failure, the drug adverse effects on the gastro-intestinal tract resemble symptoms due to uraemia (nausea, vomiting, anorexia, abdominal pain). Theophylline would therefore appear to be a good candidate for TDM[21]. There is, however, debate as to whether it is worthwhile with many respiratory physicians doubting its value.

One problem is that the therapeutic range is not well defined, though it is usually quoted as 10–20 ml/L. Dose-related adverse effects are not uncommon with concentrations at the upper end of the 'therapeutic range'. Also, many patients appear to have good control of their respiratory problems with concentrations which would be reported as subtherapeutic. It is possible to measure a dynamic end point in the form of either formal pulmonary function tests in the laboratory or peak expiratory flow rate in the clinic. This measure of dynamic end point is of value in ensuring optimum treatment. However, it is not always helpful in deciding on dose changes in a symptomatic patient. Many non-drug factors affect the measured airways resistance, such that it is difficult to get a good correlation between plasma drug concentration and response.

Since theophylline exhibits saturation kinetics, it is essential to measure the plasma drug concentration before giving an intravenous dose to an acutely dyspnoeic patient who has been taking regular theophylline medication. Toxic effects are common when intravenous theophylline is given to such patients without first checking blood levels. Clearly, it is important to have an assay method available for instant use and which will give a result in a short time. Few could argue with the value of TDM in the acute situation.

The value of TDM for theophylline in adjusting doses on a less acute basis is not entirely clear. As in the management of epilepsy, it would seem reasonable to check the blood concentration if the patient is still having symptoms despite an apparently adequate dose. The drug cannot be labelled ineffective unless it has been demonstrated that there was a satisfactory blood concentration. TDM is also of value in differentiating poor compliance from low levels due to rapid theophylline clearance if further samples are taken following dose adjustment. Concentration measurement can also be useful in preventing toxicity in patients who are well controlled. If the drug level is around the upper end of the target range, it may be possible to reduce the dose to minimize the risk of adverse effects without loss of efficacy. Apart from the similarity of uraemic symptoms mentioned above, there are no specific problems with theophylline TDM in renal failure as theophylline is not extensively bound (60%) and is eliminated by hepatic metabolism.

There is less experience of individual dose prediction methods with theophylline than for digoxin and phenytoin. However, computer programs to aid dose adjustment are available. Evaluation of one program showed a large initial dose prediction error but, if one concentration measurement was used, the prediction was good and could be further improved if two concentrations were measured[17]. Further experience and evaluation of these methods is necessary. A particular problem with theophylline is the large number of conventional and slow-release formulations which are becoming available. Timing of samples is important and the optimum time may vary depending on the product used and the frequency of dosing.

Cyclosporin

Cyclosporin is a relatively new immunosuppressive drug which prolongs allograft survival without depression of bone marrow[22]. The major problem is that it may produce dose-dependent nephrotoxicity. Since cyclosporin has a narrow therapeutic index and is at risk of damaging the organ it is supposed to protect following renal transplantation, there has been considerable interest in monitoring blood cyclosporin concentrations. The dynamic end points, such as creatinine clearance, are not reliable for titration of dose as a decrease in creatinine clearance could indicate either graft rejection due to inadequate immunosuppression or toxicity due to excessive dosage.

Cyclosporin is extensively metabolized in the liver with over 25 metabolites identified. At least three of the metabolites have immunosuppressive activity *in vitro*. One of these (M17) is a major metabolite. Inducers of the hepatic mixed function oxidase drug metabolizing enzymes (phenobarbitone, rifampicin) may reduce cyclosporin-induced renal dysfunction. This could be due either to more rapid clearance of the parent drug or diversion of metabolism away from a pathway which could produce toxic intermediate metabolites. Phenytoin also lowers cyclosporin concentrations but it has been suggested that this is due to reduced absorption rather than enzyme induction[23].

TDM for cycloporin should be considered because:

(1) There is wide interindividual variation in its pharmacokinetics. Kinetics are affected by age, disease state, other drugs and type of transplant.
(2) A minimum concentration is necessary to prevent rejection.
(3) Major toxicity is dose related and trough concentrations should be maintained below the level at which adverse effects are likely.
(4) Non-compliance is an important cause of graft loss after 60 days.

There is debate regarding the blood concentration levels necessary both for effective treatment and toxicity. Much of the debate may be due to poor assay methods or sampling techniques.

The main problem is developing a reliable assay method suitable for routine use. A radioimmunoassay kit is available and attempts have been made to develop HPLC methods. Methods using polyclonal antibodies for radioimmunoassay show cross reaction with some of the metabolites. Concentrations of 'cyclosporin' are reported as higher using this method than with HPLC. It has been suggested that the active M17 metabolite is one of those which cross reacts. This clearly makes it difficult to interpret results which are said to be measurements of total parent drug concentration. Monoclonal antibody will give a more selective measurement of parent cyclosporin concentration but some cross reactivity is still possible[24]. High performance liquid chromatography is relatively specific for parent drug in a good system but it is still possible for metabolites to co-elute with parent drug. The ultimate answer is to use mass spectrometry but this does not lend itself to routine clinical use. Drug concentrations reported therefore depend on the analytical method used. In addition, the body fluid used is important. Whole blood, serum and plasma give different results. Concentrations of cyclosporin in whole blood are approximately double those in plasma because of distribution of cyclosporin into erthyrocytes. This distribution is dependent on temperature of separation, haematocrit and drug concentration. It is, therefore, preferable to use whole blood because the results are more reproducible. The 'therapeutic range' used must be suitable for both the analytical procedure and the body fluid used in each laboratory. It may also vary in relation to time after transplantation. There is agreement that, at least, very low levels or very high levels are useful to distinguish rejection from nephrotoxicity.

Initial doses are usually 10–20 mg/kg daily by the oral route or 2.5–5 mg/kg daily by intravenous infusion. An oral dose would be reduced to 6–8 mg/kg daily by day 6 with a further reduction to 5–6 mg/kg by day 180 post transplant. The dose selected depends on the patient's age, transplant type, concurrent disease and concomitant drug therapy. The dose may then be adjusted after considering the initial response to therapy, the clinical and biochemical state of the patient and the cyclosporin blood concentrations. Cyclosporin concentrations should be measured twice weekly initially, decreasing to monthly when conditions are stable. It has been suggested that smaller initial doses (1 mg/kg daily for 2 days by intravenous infusion), with an increase according to blood concentrations when the renal graft is functioning well, would reduce long-term nephrotoxicity. Early results found no difference up to 90 days post transplant when the low-dose regime was compared with conventional dosing. Long-term outcome results are awaited. For renal transplant, the lower end of the target range is a trough whole blood concentration of 100 μg/L. The upper end used varies from 200–400 μg/L depending on transplant centre but these ranges must be regarded as provisional and may be modified with further experience.

Drug Overdose

TDM with accurate and repeated blood drug concentration measurements is not usually necessary for most drugs following overdose. In most cases, simple colorimetric tests are sufficient to identify drugs which might have been taken or to confirm ingestion of drugs known to be in the patient's possession. Colorimetric tests are highly susceptible to interference from closely related drugs and endogenous compounds. Attempts have been made to develop rapid screening methods with improved specificity using chromatography but such methods are not widely available.

However, in some situations, it is important to obtain an accurate concentration measurement using a specific analytical procedure. Examples are paracetamol, aspirin, phenytoin and phenobarbitone. The aim of TDM in this situation is to quantify the initial drug level and obtain an estimate of the drug clearance by repeat concentration measurement so that specific treatment may be instituted and the effects monitored by further concentration measurements.

The place of paracetamol concentration measurement is well established. If treatment with *N*-acetylcysteine is to be instituted, it should begin, ideally, within 10 h of drug ingestion. A very high initial level (200 mg/L at 4 h post drug ingestion) or slow rate of decline, so that the concentration is likely to be above 50 mg/L at 12 h post ingestion, is predictive of likely liver damage and the need for prophylactic treatment. Samples should be taken as early as possible so that the laboratory can measure the concentration and report the result well within the ten-hour period for optimal therapeutic benefit. Paracetamol exerts its main toxic effects on the liver and kidney. In patients with pre-existing renal disease, there is no additional difficulty in interpreting the plasma concentration measurements. However, such patients may be at increased risk of renal and hepatic damage and it is essential to consider the need for *N*-acetylcysteine at an early stage and, if the levels are borderline, it is prudent to give the antidote where it might not be strictly necessary in patients with normal renal function.

Aspirin and phenobarbitone concentration measurements are necessary to decide on the need for forced diuresis or dialysis. Serial aspirin measurements are more useful than a single sample because of a prolonged phase of absorption following large overdose. Forced alkaline diuresis needs to be considered if the salicylate level is greater than 500 mg/L. In very severe poisoning, with levels greater than 900 mg/L, patients should be considered for haemodialysis or haemoperfusion. Decisions regarding such treatment need to be made at an early stage before the patient becomes moribund. Similarly, with phenobarbitone, serial measurements are helpful to decide if alkaline diuresis (serum level > 75 mg/L) or dialysis (serum level > 100 mg/L) are indicated to reduce the risk of organ damage and the time spent on a ventilator. In the presence of pre-existing renal disease, it is clearly unwise to rely on alkaline diuresis and patients should be considered for dialysis at lower serum levels because their rate of drug elimination will be slower than in patients with normal renal function.

Phenytoin overdose is an unusual situation. Following massive overdose, the plasma concentrations do not reach enormous peaks but plateau at around 60–100 mg/L and stay elevated for up to 14 days before starting to decline. The mechanism for this phenomenon is not completely understood. However, daily concentration measurements are advisable to give a guide to when improvement in the clinical condition is likely to begin. Full supportive care is necessary until the concentrations begin to fall. The special problems of interpreting phenytoin concentrations in the presence of renal failure have been discussed above. There are no cases of massive phenytoin overdose in patients with pre-existing renal disease in the literature. It is, therefore, not known whether such patients will also show a prolonged plateau phase.

Compliance with drug therapy

TDM on a routine basis cannot be recommended for the vast majority of drugs. The main problems are that most drugs do not have a clearly defined therapeutic range of plasma drug concentration and the cost of the procedure could not be justified in terms of the likely benefit.

Measuring an occasional drug concentration can be useful in the evaluation of failure to respond to drug treatment in selected patients. Poor compliance with drug therapy is an important clinical problem. This is particularly true in the elderly and patients on multiple drug treatment. It is clearly unjust wrongly to accuse patients of not taking their drugs. If patients give an assurance, on diplomatic questioning, that they are taking their therapy, it is worth considering measurement of a blood drug concentration to try to establish the true situation. In the first instance, a random clinic sample is sufficient. If the level is low, this does not confirm non-compliance. Alternative explanations are poor drug absorption or unusually rapid excretion. A second sample should be taken at a suitable time following the administration of a dose of the drug under close supervision. A low level of the second sample indicates a pharmacokinetic problem, but, if this level is in the 'therapeutic range', the suspicion of non-compliance is confirmed. Many patients are helped to respond better to treatment after discussion of their compliance problem. An alternative approach to this problem is to administer a small dose of a marker substance with the patient's drug and measure the marker in blood. Recent studies claim that a small dose of phenobarbitone is useful in this situation but further evaluation is necessary[25]. Some examples of non-compliance have been discussed above with drugs suitable for TDM. The role of occasional concentration measurements can be illustrated by considering the use of warfarin, propranolol and tricyclic antidepressants.

Warfarin is a drug with wide variation in pharmacokinetics and a narrow therapeutic index. It satisfies most of the criteria for TDM, but, because of wide dynamic variation in the response to a given plasma concentration, it is preferable to measure a biochemical marker as an end point of the effect of warfarin on blood coagulation. The prothrombin time measurement is the standard test used, though recent evidence suggests that other end points might be more appropriate in some circumstances. Warfarin concentration measurement is useful when patients fail to respond to doses of warfarin at the upper end of the usual dose range. Some patients are genetically resistant to warfarin or may be resistant because of other factors such as drug therapy (e.g. phenobarbitone). Warfarin measurements allow the rare condition of genetic resistance to be identified and distinguished from poor compliance.

Propranolol is a lipid-soluble β-adrenoceptor antagonist with extensive first-pass metabolism. This results in very wide variation in blood concentrations following oral dosing. It is, however, rarely necessary to measure propranolol concentrations because the therapeutic index is relatively wide and the pulse rate can be used as a guide to dose adjustment. Patients with greater than average first-pass effect require more drug to achieve a good clinical response. Blood concentrations would be low in both these patients and patients with poor compliance. However, administration of a supervised oral dose should result in higher levels in the non-compliant patient but no change in patients with high first pass.

TDM is available for tricyclic antidepressants in some centres. They are not ideal drugs for TDM because the therapeutic range is not well defined, metabolites are active and protein binding is variable. Some of these problems do also apply to drugs such as carbamazepine but most authorities do not feel that there is enough benefit to justify routine tricyclic concentration monitoring. One of the difficulties in treating depression is that there is a delay of 1–2 weeks until a response can be observed. If the initial dose chosen is too low for the individual patient, then a further delay in response will occur after dose adjustment. Measuring blood levels may, therefore, be useful to exclude poor compliance with therapy and to detect patients with low steady-state concentrations. There is considerable scope for improving drug treatment of depression but TDM cannot be of major benefit until assay methods which routinely measure free concentrations of parent drug and active metabolites are available. Such methods must, then, be fully evaluated in general clinical use.

Cost-effectiveness

Audit of use of the TDM service has been carried out in several laboratories. The general conclusion is that the standard of use of drug concentration measurements is poor, but that it can be improved by intervention of staff with a special interest in TDM to recommend dose alterations. Such a service requires funding, with the main component being salaries to cover technical staff to perform the drug assays and clinical biochemists, pharmacists or clinical pharmacologists to report the results and recommend appropriate dose changes. In addition, there is a large initial outlay to cover analytical equipment, preferably with computer facilities, and running costs for materials. TDM services compete with other services for funding and attempts have been made to establish whether or not TDM is cost-effective. Such studies are notoriously difficult to perform as the benefits of TDM and other services are difficult to quantify in terms of financial cost. There is very little information available on cost-benefit analysis of TDM and there are no controlled prospective studies of cost-effectiveness[26].

Beneficial effects of TDM may be direct or indirect.

Direct benefits are:

(1) Improved efficacy – increased survival, reduced length of hospital stay, increased patient well being.
(2) Reduced adverse effects with reduced costs of treating these.
(3) Reduced costs to patient – fewer clinic visits, less time off work.
(4) Contribution to the community – increased productivity, less time off work.

Indirect benefits are:

(1) Education of the physician to improve general prescribing.
(2) Improved patient compliance because of better understanding of treatment.
(3) Pharmacokinetic data available for research on large populations.

TDM cannot be cost-effective unless it is used properly. It is not sufficient simply to have an assay service available without appropriate feedback. Such a system results in about 50% of samples being taken at inappropriate times. About 50% of correctly timed samples are wrongly interpreted or not acted upon. Significant improvement has been shown to follow implementation of a more active reporting system using request forms designed for TDM and reports which recommend appropriate dose changes[17]. The type of benefit to be expected from improved use of individual drugs has been discussed above. Prospective studies of the cost-effectiveness of an active TDM service should be carried out, though some of the benefits and costs are difficult to quantify. In patients with renal failure, the extra costs of TDM are small in comparison with the overall cost of treating renal failures and its complications. For drugs, such as gentamicin, digoxin and phenytoin, the expected benefits are likely to be greater than in the general population because the risks of adverse effects are higher.

Pharmacodynamics

TDM with adjustment of the drug dose to achieve a concentration within the desired target range only allows for inter-individual variation in drug disposition. Variation in response may also occur due to differences in receptor sensitivity. Both the therapeutic effect and adverse effects will occur at different plasma concentrations in different patients.

In order to monitor a drug effect, it is clearly essential that the response to it can be objectively measured. This is easier if there is a good relationship between drug dose and response and where the dose-response curve is neither too steep nor too flat.

For some drugs, there is a clinical effect which can be measured relatively easily using non-invasive methods. Examples are blood pressure for antihypertensive drugs, ventricular rate for digoxin in the treatment of atrial fibrillation and ocular pressure for drugs used to treat glaucoma. Other drugs can be monitored because they alter a biochemical parameter which can be readily measured in a sample of blood or urine. Examples are blood sugar measurements for controlling hypoglycaemic drugs, prothrombin time measurement for warfarin and serum urate for drugs used in the treatment of gout.

Unfortunately, for many drugs, the response is more difficult to quantify or there may be an excessive lag period between dosage alteration and a measurable change in response. The treatment of depression is a good example of both of these problems. Although the degree of depression can be documented, the measurements used are subjective and show wide intra-individual variation. Also, there is a delay of up to 3 weeks before drug treatment begins to be effective. A further example is the use of corticosteroids to suppress inflammation. There is no clear dose–response relationship and, inevitably, there is a delay between giving the drug and observing an improvement. Nevertheless, it is possible to consider a limited scheme of monitoring provided the limitations are recognized. Monitoring in this situation requires testing for adverse effects while keeping the dose below the level at which problems arise. With corticosteroids, blood glucose and serum potassium measurements are helpful. Many drug effects which cannot be objectively measured with available techniques will become accessible to measurement in the future.

Drug use is often difficult because of wide interindividual variation in the response to a given dose. Most drugs are still prescribed using a 'best guess' approach. This works reasonably well if the drug has a wide therapeutic range and a low incidence of adverse effects. The presence of renal failure may increase the risk of problems. If no suitable end point can be measured, consideration should be given to modifying the usual dose to allow for the effect of renal disease.

Pharmacodynamic monitoring is also essential to detect drug adverse effects at an early stage. This is particularly important for drugs which cause renal impairment. The effect on renal function is often reversible if it is detected at an early stage. Consideration must therefore be given to the use of regular tests of renal function for drugs known to cause renal damage.

Monitoring of renal function is clearly easier than for most other organs since urine is readily accessible for measurement of creatinine, protein and enzymes. In addition, measurement of serum creatinine gives a more reliable guide to functional changes than is available in failure of other organs, such as the liver.

Creatinine clearance, calculated using a blood sample and timed urine sample, is the most useful widely-available simple test for repeated monitoring of function. However, there are often problems in obtaining a reliable timed urine collection, particularly in elderly out-patients. A formula for calculating creatinine clearance using serum creatinine, body weight and age has been devised[27].

$$C_{cr}(\mathrm{ml\,min^{-1}}) = \frac{(140 - \text{age})\ (\text{weight in kg})}{72 \times \text{serum creatinine}\ (\mathrm{mg\,dl^{-1}})}$$

In a study of 129 patients, this formula was found to be reliable except in small adults (<45 kg) and pregnant women[28]. The authors feel that it is better than serum creatinine alone when adjustment of drug dose is required in renal failure. The nomograms for calculating digoxin and gentamicin dosage are based on the three factors used in the calculation (age, weight, serum creatinine).

The angiotensin converting enzyme (ACE) inhibitors, such as captopril and enalapril, are being increasingly used in the treatment of hypertension and cardiac failure. Both drugs may cause renal failure, particularly in the elderly and in patients with renal artery stenosis. Regular monitoring of serum creatinine or creatinine clearance is essential to detect the development of renal impairment at an early stage[29]. Although renal failure may occur after prolonged treatment with ACE inhibitors, it usually occurs within a few months of starting treatment. Creatinine should therefore be measured several times within the first six months of treatment. The need for longer term monitoring is less certain but it would be prudent to monitor renal function every 6–12 months until more information on long-term safety becomes available. Serum creatinine usually returns to pretreatment values after stopping ACE inhibitors. Other drugs which cause renal failure should also be considered for monitoring in this way.

Urinary protein excretion is useful for monitoring drugs which might cause nephrotic syndrome or in monitoring the response to treatment of nephrotic syndrome. A screening stick-based test is suitable in the first instance. However, if significant proteinuria is detected, a quantitative assessment should be made on a 24-hour urine collection. Proteinuria occurs in up to 19% of patients treated with gold for rheumatoid arthritis. Around 10–30% of these patients develop nephrotic syndrome[30]. The onset of proteinuria is not related to the duration of treatment or total amount of gold administered. Unfortunately, the proteinuria is not reversible in all cases in the short term but has been reported to resolve eventually (up to 39 months) if the gold is stopped[31]. Monitoring serum gold levels is of no value but a urine sample should be tested for protein at monthly intervals. Similar regular follow up is also necessary for penicillamine.

There is considerable interest in the use of urinary enzyme measurements in the diagnosis and prediction of drug-induced renal damage. The three-day excretion pattern of urinary alanine aminopeptidase (AAP) has been reported to be of value in assessing the nephrotoxic potential of gentamicin in human volunteers. However, urinary AAP measurement did not predict gentamicin toxicity when it was used in seriously ill patients[32]. AAP is a brush border enzyme. When the lysosomal enzyme *N*-acetylglucosaminidase (NAG) was studied it was found to predict gentamicin toxicity[33]. Urinary NAG concentrations before gentamicin treatment and the excretion pattern during treatment were both claimed to be of value in predicting nephrotoxicity. A third group of urinary enzymes are low-molecular-weight enzymes which are excreted by glomerular filtration. One of these enzymes, β_2-microglobulin has been studied but there is no agreement as to its value in demonstrating drug-induced nephrotoxicity[28]. NAG is the most promising of the urinary enzyme measurements. However, it is not yet generally available for routine use. Measurement of NAG will need to be compared with serum creatinine measurement to determine which is best for individual drugs.

CONCLUSION

Therapeutic drug monitoring has a limited, though important, role to play in the overall strategy for drug use in renal disease. For a small number of drugs, TDM is essential to help minimize problems, both of subtherapeutic dosing and adverse effects. Future development of assay methods to measure free drug will make the interpretation of drug concentration measurements easier in the presence of renal failure. A more active TDM service with recommendations for dose changes and follow up would help to improve patient care, though formal evidence of cost-effectiveness is lacking. As with any other laboratory investigation, the results obtained should always be interpreted with respect to the complete clinical picture. Drug concentration measurement cannot allow for variation in the dynamic response and therefore is of little benefit where a dynamic end point can be measured. The encouragement of rational drug therapy through TDM has benefits for the use of other drugs not normally considered suitable for TDM. This indirect educational benefit is often overlooked when discussing the benefits of TDM. The education process will be further helped by the development of improved nomograms or computer programs to aid the prescriber in making the choice of initial dose and dose adjustment in conjunction with measurement of serum drug concentration.

REFERENCES

1. Scott, A. K. and Hawksworth, G. M. (1981). Drug absorption. *Br. Med. J.*, **282,** 462–463
2. Bennet, W. M. (1986). The kidney and drug pharmacokinetics. In Bennet, W. M. (ed.) *Drugs and Renal Disease*. (Edinburgh: Churchill Livingstone)
3. Bateman, D. N., Gokal, R., Dodd, T. R. P. and Blain, P. G. (1981). The pharmacokinetics of single doses of metoclopramide in renal failure. *Eur. J. Clin. Pharmacol.*, **19,** 437–441
4. Aitio, M.-L. and Vuorenmaa, T. (1980). Enhanced metabolism and diminished

efficacy of disopyramide by enzyme induction? *Br. J. Clin. Pharmacol.*, **9,** 149–152

5. Nemeth, I. and Szeleczki, T. (1981). Enhanced drug metabolism and renal dysfunction. *Br. J. Clin. Pharmacol.*, **11,** 92–93
6. Bridgeman, J. F., Rosen, S. M. and Thorp, J. M. (1972). Complications during clofibrate treatment of nephrotic syndrome hyperlipoproteinaemia. *Lancet*, **2,** 506–509
7. Erill, S. and Calvo, R. (1986). Qualitative changes of proteins as a cause of altered drug binding in serum. In Tillement, J.-P. and Lindenlaub, E. (eds.) *Protein Binding and Drug Transport*, pp. 337–348. (Stuttgart/New York: F. K. Schattauer Verlag)
8. Lindup, W. E., Bishop, K. A. and Collier, R. (1986). Drug binding defect of uraemic plasma: contribution of endogenous binding inhibitors. In Tillement, J.-P. and Lindenlaub, E. (eds.) *Protein Binding and Drug Transport*, pp. 397–414. (Stuttgart/New York: F. K. Schattauer Verlag)
9. Kato, R. (1977). Drug metabolism under pathological and abnormal physiological states in animals and man. *Xenobiotica*, **7,** 25–92
10. Ochs, H. R., Greenblatt, D. J., Kaschell, J. H., Klehr, U., Divoll, M. and Abernethy, D. J. (1981). Diazepam kinetics in patients with renal insufficiency or hyperthyroidism. *Br. J. Clin. Pharmacol.*, **12,** 829–832
11. Barnes, J. N., Williams, A. J., Tomson, M. J. F., Toseland, P. A. and Goodwin, F. J. (1985). Dihydrocodeine in renal failure: further evidence for an important role of the kidney in the handling of opioid drugs. *Br. Med. J.*, **290,** 740–742
12. Verbeeck, R. K., Branch, R. A. and Wilkinson, G. R. (1981). Drug metabolism in renal failure: pharmacokinetic and clinical implications. *Clin. Pharmacokin.*, **6,** 329–345
13. Osborne, R. J., Joel, S. P. and Slevin, M. L. (1986). Morphine intoxication in renal failure: the role of morphine-6-glucuronide. *Br. Med. J.*, **292,** 1548–1549
14. MacKichan, J. J., Duffner, P. K. and Cohen, M. E. (1981). Salivary concentrations and plasma protein binding of carbamazepine and carbamazepine 10, 11 – epoxide in epileptic patients. *Br. J. Clin. Pharmacol.*, **12,** 31–37
15. Johnston, G. D. (1980). Digoxin dose precision: prescribing aids or intuition? *Drugs*, **20,** 494–499
16. Chennavasin, P. and Brater, D. C. (1981). Nomograms for drug use in renal disease. *Clin. Pharmacokin.*, **6,** 193–214
17. Whiting, B., Bryson, S. M., Derkx, F. H. M., Thomson, A. H., Fotheringham, G. H. and Joel, S. E. (1984). Clinical pharmacokinetics: a comprehensive system for therapeutic drug monitoring and prescribing. *Br. Med. J.*, **288,** 541–545
18. Barza, M. and Lauermann, M. (1978). Why monitor serum levels of digoxin? *Clin Pharmacokin.*, **3,** 202–215
19. Richens, A. (1979). Clinical pharmacokinetics of phenytoin. *Clin. Pharmacokin.*, **4,** 153–169
20. Richens, A. and Dunlop, A. (1975). Serum phenytoin levels in the management of epilepsy. *Lancet*, **2,** 247–248
21. Hendeles, L., Weinberger, M. and Johnson, G. (1978). Monitoring serum theophylline levels. *Clin. Pharmacokin.*, **3,** 294–312
22. Ptachcinski, R. J., Venkataraman, R. and Burckart, G. J. (1986). Clinical pharmacokinetics of cyclosporin. *Clin. Pharmacokin.*, **11,** 107–132
23. Rowland, M. and Gupta, S. K. (1987). Cyclosporin–phenytoin interaction: re-

evaluation using metabolite data. *Br. J. Clin. Pharmacol.*, **24,** 329–334

24. Quesniaux, V., Tees, R., Schreier, M. H., Maurer, G. and van Regenmortel, M. H. V. (1987). Potential of monoclonal antibodies to improve therapeutic monitoring of cyclosporine. *Clin. Chem.*, **33,** 32–37
25. Feely, M., Cooke, J., Price, D., Singleton, S., Mehta, A., Bradford, L. and Calvert, R. (1987). Low-dose phenobarbitone as an indicator of compliance with drug therapy. *Br. J. Clin. Pharmacol.*, **24,** 77–83
26. Vozeh, S. (1987). Cost-effectiveness of therapeutic drug monitoring. *Clin. Pharmacokin.*, **13,** 131–140
27. Cockcroft, D. W. and Gault, M. H. (1976). Prediction of creatinine clearance from serum creatinine. *Nephron*, **16,** 31–41
28. Porter, G. A. (1986). Renal function tests. In Bennet, W. M. (ed.) *Drugs and Renal Disease*, pp. 1–17. (Edinburgh: Churchill Livingstone)
29. Breckenridge, A. (1988). Angiotensin converting enzyme inhibitors. *Br. Med. J.*, **296,** 618–620
30. Collins, A. J. (1987). Gold treatment for rheumatoid arthritis: reassurance on proteinuria. *Br. Med. J.*, **295,** 739–740
31. Hall, C. L. Fothergill, N. J., Blackwell, M. M., Harrison, P. R., MacKenzie, J. C. and MacIver, A. G. (1987). The natural course of gold nephropathy: long term study of 21 patients. *Br. Med. J.*, **295,** 745–748
32. Davey, P. G., Geddes, A. M. and Cawley, D. M. (1983). Study of alanine aminopeptidase excretion as a test of gentamicin nephrotoxicity. *J. Antimic. Chemother.*, **11,** 455–465
33. Gibey, R., Dupond, J. L., Alber, D., des Floris, R. L. and Henry, J.-C. (1981). Predictive value of urinary *N*-acetyl-beta-D-glucosamine (NAG), alanine aminopeptidase (AAP) and beta-2-microglobulin (β_2M) in evaluating nephrotoxicity of gentamicin. *Clin. Chim. Acta*, **116,** 25–34

INDEX

GPSR Compliance

The European Union's (EU) General Product Safety Regulation (GPSR) is a set of rules that requires consumer products to be safe and our obligations to ensure this.

If you have any concerns about our products, you can contact us on ProductSafety@springernature.com

In case Publisher is established outside the EU, the EU authorized representative is:

Springer Nature Customer Service Center GmbH
Europaplatz 3
69115 Heidelberg, Germany

Batch number: 10607224

Printed by Printforce, the Netherlands